Adult Gerontology Acute Care Nurse Practitioner Certification

- ▮ **Note-Taking Techniques:** Discover various methods for taking effective and organized notes during lectures or while reading textbooks.
- ●**Critical Thinking Skills:** Develop your ability to analyze, evaluate, and synthesize information to make informed decisions and solve problems.
- ⏰ **Time Blocking and the Pomodoro Technique:** Learn about time management techniques like time blocking and the Pomodoro Technique to enhance productivity
- 🎐 **Stress Relief Strategies:** Overcome exam anxiety with mindfulness, relaxation exercises, and mental resilience techniques.
- ▮ **Practice Makes Perfect:** Explore the importance of practice exams, sample questions, and mock tests, and understand how to analyze your performance to identify areas for improvement.
- ● **Test-Taking Tactics:** Master the art of answering different types of questions, managing your time during the exam, and maintaining focus under pressure.

The following is a disclaimer of liability:

The goal of this book is to provide the reader with background information on the numerous topics that are discussed throughout the book. It is offered for sale with the understanding that neither the author nor the publisher are engaged in the practice of providing professional advice of any type, including but not limited to advice pertaining to legal matters, medical matters, or other matters. In the event that one need the aid of a professional, one must seek the assistance of an experienced professional who is qualified to provide it.

This book has been laboriously labored over in an effort to make it as accurate as is humanly feasible, and it has taken a lot of labor. However, there is a possibility that there are inaccuracies, both in the typography and the actual content of the article. The author and publisher of this book do not accept any responsibility or liability to any third party for any loss or damage caused, or represented to have been caused, directly or indirectly, by the information that is included in this book. This rule applies to any loss or harm that may have been caused, or is suspected of having been caused, by the information that is presented in this book.

This information is provided "as is," without any guarantees or warranties regarding its completeness, accuracy, usefulness, or timeliness. The information is presented "as is" without any guarantees or warranties of any kind. The reader is highly encouraged to seek the opinion of a certified expert or professionals in the field in order to obtain the most up-to-date knowledge that is currently available.

information and compiled data.

In no way, shape, or form does the viewpoints or policies of any specific organisation or professional body come over in this book in any kind whatsoever. Any slights that could be interpreted as being directed toward specific individuals or groups were not intended, despite the fact that they may have occurred.

TABLE OF CONTENT

STUDY GUIDE

Introduction

The Role of the Adult-Gerontology Acute Care Nurse Practitioner
Purpose and Importance of Certification

Chapter 1: The AG-ACNP Certification Exam

Understanding the Certification Exam
Preparing for the Certification Exam
Test-Taking Strategies

Chapter 2: Review of Core Clinical Concepts

Cardiovascular System
Pulmonary System
Neurological System
Gastrointestinal System
Renal and Urinary Systems
Hematological and Immune Systems

Chapter 3: Advanced Clinical Assessment

Health History and Physical Examination
Diagnostic Tests and Procedures
Data Analysis and Interpretation

Chapter 4: Diagnostic Reasoning

Differential Diagnosis
Clinical Decision-Making
Evidence-Based Practice

Chapter 5: Acute and Chronic Conditions

Cardiac and Vascular Conditions
Respiratory Conditions
Neurological Conditions
Gastrointestinal Conditions
Renal and Urinary Conditions
Hematological Conditions
Endocrine and Metabolic Conditions

Chapter 6: Pharmacology and Medication Management

Principles of Pharmacotherapy
Common Medications in AG-ACNP Practice
Medication Management and Patient Education

Chapter 7: Management of Acute and Critical Care Patients

Critical Care Concepts
Advanced Life Support
Care of the Postoperative Patient
Multisystem Complications

Chapter 8: Healthcare Systems and Policy

Healthcare Delivery Models
Legal and Ethical Issues
Healthcare Policy and Advocacy

Chapter 9: Professional Development

Lifelong Learning
Continuing Education

Networking and Mentorship

Chapter 10: Preparing for Success

Study Plans and Resources
Test-Taking Strategies
Managing Test Anxiety

Chapter 11: The Certification Journey

Application and Registration
Test Day and Beyond
Receiving Your Certification

Chapter 12: Gerontological Care

Understanding the Aging Process
Special Considerations for Geriatric Patients
Common Geriatric Syndromes

Chapter 13: Wound Care and Procedures

Assessment and Management of Wounds
Advanced Wound Care Techniques
Invasive Procedures in Acute Care

Chapter 14: Pulmonary Management

Mechanical Ventilation
Respiratory Failure
Chronic Obstructive Pulmonary Disease (COPD) Management

Chapter 15: Cardiac Rhythm Interpretation

ECG Basics
Arrhythmia Recognition and Management
Cardiac Monitoring in Acute Care

Chapter 16: Advanced Practice Procedures

Central Line Insertion
Thoracentesis and Paracentesis
Arterial Line Insertion

Chapter 17: Patient and Family Education

Effective Communication
Health Literacy
Engaging Patients and Families in Care

Chapter 18: Quality Improvement and Patient Safety

Identifying and Addressing Medical Errors
Quality Improvement Initiatives
Safety Protocols in Acute Care

The Beginning of a New Era in Adult-Gerontology Acute Care Nursing: Paving the Path to Excellence in Nursing

The work of the Adult-Gerontology Acute Care Nurse Practitioner (AG-ACNP) is a shining example of excellence in the field of healthcare, which places a premium on accuracy, expertise, and compassionate treatment of patients. AG-ACNPs are at the vanguard of an ever-changing healthcare landscape because they are committed to providing advanced care to adult and geriatric patients who are coping with acute and complex health difficulties. To engage on the path to becoming a certified AG-ACNP is to undertake a journey that requires devotion, a commitment to continual learning, and a dedication to improve the results for patients. This book, "Mastering Adult-Gerontology Acute Care Nurse Practitioner Certification," will guide you along this route to excellence and assist you in overcoming the challenges that are still in front of you.

The AG-ACNP: A Shining Example of Superiority

Being a healthcare provider is only one aspect of an AG-ACNP's responsibilities; they also have the need to provide an example of superior performance in their profession. AG-ACNPs are advanced practice registered nurses who have specialized in acute care. They manage the healthcare needs of adult and elderly patients who have complex conditions that often pose a threat to their lives. They act as advocates, diagnosticians, and carers for patients, making certain that patients receive the highest quality of care throughout the times in their lives when they are at their most vulnerable.

The expertise of an AG-ACNP combines sophisticated clinical assessment, diagnostic reasoning, pharmacology knowledge, and the management of complex medical diseases. This gives them a skill set that is truly unique. They are prepared to work in a wide range of healthcare settings, including critical care units, emergency departments, cardiology and respiratory units, as well as other settings. This challenging position calls for an in-depth comprehension of critical thinking, advanced clinical abilities, and a dedication to the application of evidence-based practice.

However, what distinguishes the AG-ACNP from other nurse practitioners is their commitment to provide holistic care to patients throughout the entirety of their health journey. AG-ACNPs are there every step of the way to ensure that patients receive the care and attention they require, whether it be managing chronic diseases, stabilizing acute crises, or aiding patients and their families in making decisions on end-of-life care.

The Essential Path to Acquiring Certification

Becoming certified as an AG-ACNP is a noteworthy accomplishment that demonstrates one's dedication to achieving the highest possible standards in nursing. Certification is not simply a piece of paper or a set of letters after your name; it is a mark of your dedication, your competence, and your preparedness to meet the challenges and complexities of the healthcare environment head on. Certification is not just a piece of paper or a set of letters after your name. It is the fulfillment of a lifelong ambition to have a significant influence on the lives of patients and to take part in a profession that is well regarded and esteemed.

This book is intended to serve as your reliable guide on the path toward earning this essential certification. It is a wonderful resource for nurse practitioner students, practicing nurse practitioners who are working toward becoming AG-ACNPs, and even experienced healthcare professionals who are eager to increase their expertise in adult-gerontology acute care nursing. This book will give you with the knowledge and tactics you need to thrive in your certification path and deliver great care to adult and geriatric patients in acute care settings. It will do so by providing you with content that is comprehensive, guidance from experts, and insights into the practical application of those insights.

The First Step in the Process: Taking the AG-ACNP Certification Exam

An essential first step for any healthcare practitioner who is interested in obtaining their AG-ACNP certification is to have a fundamental understanding of the certification exam. The certification exam is a strenuous evaluation of your knowledge and clinical skills. It covers a wide variety of topics that are necessary for practicing medicine in a manner that is both safe and successful in acute care settings. This book will provide you with a clear idea of what to anticipate and how to prepare for the certification exam by delving into the fundamental principles and clinical competencies that will be assessed.

The process of studying for this certification exam can be both exciting and intimidating, regardless of whether you are a recent nursing school graduate, an experienced nurse, or someone who is returning to nursing practice. We will walk you through the steps of registering for the exam, maximizing the effectiveness of your studying, and establishing strategies for the test itself. On the day of the exam, we will discuss tried-and-true methods for overcoming test anxiety and performing to your full potential. As you work toward your ultimate goal of becoming a certified AG-ACNP, you may look to this book as a reliable companion along the way.

How to Make Your Way Through the Complex Clinical Landscape

The nursing profession is one that is always evolving, and when it comes to acute care for adults and older adults, the breadth and depth of clinical knowledge can be very overwhelming. In order to successfully traverse this intricate environment, we will investigate a wide range of issues, beginning with a discussion of fundamental clinical ideas. A crucial aspect of AG-ACNP practice is the acquisition of knowledge regarding the cardiovascular, pulmonary, neurological, gastrointestinal, renal, hematological, and immunological systems. In the following pages, we will not only discuss the anatomy and physiology, but we will also go into common diseases and ailments that you are likely to come across in acute care settings. These settings include hospitals, emergency rooms, and other medical facilities.

In addition to focusing on clinical review, we will place a strong emphasis on advanced clinical assessment, which is an important ability for AG-ACNPs to possess. Understanding how to properly take a patient's medical history, do a physical exam, and interpret the results of diagnostic tests and procedures is absolutely necessary for correctly diagnosing and treating complex medical disorders. In this section, we will provide you some pointers on how to collect important patient data, how to conduct reliable evaluations, and how to interpret clinical findings so that you can create a differential diagnosis.

The realm of diagnostic thinking will also be a part of our travels for us to experience. At the core of advanced practice nursing is the capacity to engage in critical thinking, perform data analysis, and arrive at evidence-based clinical judgments. We will discuss the complexities of clinical decision-making, the nuances of differential diagnosis, and the importance of evidence-based practice. This journey is not only about memorizing; rather, it is about understanding the "why" behind clinical decisions and embracing a holistic approach to the care of patients.

Treatment and Management of Acute and Ongoing Conditions

You will be at the forefront of the management of a wide variety of medical disorders if you choose to become an AG-ACNP. Patients who require your treatment will come to you with a wide variety of health problems, many of which will be difficult to treat. In this book, we will begin an in-depth investigation of these disorders, which will be arranged according to the systems of the body.

We will delve into the complexities of diagnosing, treating, and working with multidisciplinary teams to achieve the best possible outcomes for patients suffering from a wide range of illnesses, including those affecting the cardiovascular system, the respiratory system, the gastrointestinal tract, the kidneys, the endocrine system, and more. We will equip you with the essential skills and information to design patient-specific treatment plans, which may include pharmaceutical therapies and surgical procedures as appropriate.

In addition to having a firm grasp on the clinical facets of treatment, we will also attend to the emotional and psychological requirements of patients and the families of those patients. Acute and chronic diseases frequently have deep affects on individuals and their support networks; therefore, AG-ACNPs need to be adept in delivering not only medical interventions but also the emotional support and direction that patients seek. This is because acute and chronic illnesses often have substantial consequences on individuals.

Pharmacology and the Administration of Medication

The field of pharmacology is an essential component of the AG-ACNP's clinical work. Patients who seek your care are likely to be taking a variety of drugs, each of which comes with its own individual mix of benefits, dangers, and potential side effects. We will walk you through the fundamentals of pharmacotherapy, including the mechanism of action, pharmacokinetics, and pharmacodynamics of popular drugs, as well as the potential adverse effects that may be caused by them. It is crucial to one's ability to make safe and effective judgments to have a solid understanding of how drugs work and the potential consequences they have on patient care.

The act of prescribing medications is only one component of pharmacological treatment; just as important is ensuring that patients fully understand their medication schedules and are able to successfully adhere to them. As an AG-ACNP, one of the most important responsibilities you have is to educate patients about the proper use of medications and any possible adverse effects. This book will assist you in developing your expertise in the provision of medication education to your patients, so enabling them to take an active role in their own care.

Patients in Acute and Critical Care: Management of Their Care

Patients who are in a critical condition are entrusted to the care of AG-ACNPs in settings that are classified as acute care. In this course, we will investigate the field of critical care and cover topics such as the fundamentals of mechanical ventilation, respiratory failure, and the treatment of potentially life-threatening crises. This book will provide you with the knowledge and skills necessary to care for patients during the times in their lives when they are at their most vulnerable. Being proficient in critical care is a cornerstone of AG-ACNP practice, and this book will equip you with that knowledge and skills.

In addition, we will discuss the postoperative patient, with an emphasis on the particular difficulties and factors that come into play after surgical procedures. Patients undergoing surgery frequently call for vigilant monitoring, pain management, and other measures in order to avoid problems. We will discuss the postoperative treatment that should be received as well as the steps that should be taken to guarantee a speedy recovery.

In acute care, multisystem complications can present their own unique issues, which need for extensive assessments, prompt decision-making, and collaborative efforts between interdisciplinary teams. Throughout the entirety of this book, we will stress how important it is to recognize and successfully manage circumstances that are complex.

Policies and Healthcare Delivery Systems

The AG-ACNPs work within a complicated healthcare system that is impacted by both ethical and legal concerns on a daily basis. It is crucial to one's ability to perform in a safe and effective manner to have a solid understanding of healthcare delivery models, legal requirements, and ethical frameworks.

The various modes of healthcare delivery, such as primary, secondary, and tertiary care, as well as the places in which AG-ACNPs work, such as hospitals, clinics, and specialized units, will be discussed in depth throughout this book. In this lesson, we are going to look into the legal and ethical problems that define the practice of AG-ACNPs. Some of these topics include informed consent, patient rights, and advanced directives. In addition, we will have a conversation on healthcare policy, the effects of healthcare reform, and the part that AG-ACNPs play in fighting for great care.

The Never-Ending Quest for Betterment in One's Profession

Your journey does not come to an end when you earn your certification as a healthcare professional; rather, it is just getting started. Learning new things throughout one's entire life is one of the most important aspects of nursing, and throughout this book, we will stress how important it is to keep one's education current and to advance professionally.

Learning throughout one's life entails more than just education gained in a classroom setting; it also includes keeping up with ever-evolving medical knowledge, embracing new technologies, and implementing the most recent evidence-based procedures. This book will help you cultivate a mindset of continual learning and improvement, so preparing you for the dynamic field of healthcare, which is constantly evolving.

Additionally essential to the process of professional development are the activities of networking and mentoring. We are going to talk about the importance of cultivating professional relationships, finding role models, and making contributions to the development of your industry. You will be armed with the tools necessary to succeed in the ever-changing and interconnected world of healthcare with the counsel that is presented in these pages.

Your Guide to Acquiring Certification and Being Prepared for Success

When you first start out on the path to becoming an AG-ACNP certified professional, it is essential to plan and prepare thoroughly. We will assist you in developing a study plan that is suited to both your requirements and the resources at your disposal. For the purpose of assisting you in your preparation, we will provide you with access to a wide variety of resources, such as textbooks, information found online, and practice examinations. You may encounter some difficulties on your path to certification; but, if you equip yourself with the appropriate resources and techniques, you will be able to approach the certification exam with confidence and come out on top.

This book will not only supply you with the necessary knowledge, but it will also provide you with advise on how to approach and perform well on tests. From multiple-choice questions to clinical simulations, we will investigate the most productive ways to approach the many kinds of questions that might be found on exams. In addition, we will discuss the topic of test anxiety, which is a typical problem among those who are going to take a test, and present ways to help you manage your tension and perform at your best on the day of the exam.

The Path to Certification: From the Application to the Successful Completion

The process of obtaining certification as an AG-ACNP involves a number of steps, beginning with the application and ending with achievement. We will walk you through the steps of applying for the certification exam and provide an overview of the standards and processes that must be followed. In addition, we will provide guidance on how to efficiently manage your time in the days leading up to the test and ensure that you are well-prepared on the day of the examination.

Your perseverance and effort will be rewarded the minute you are successful in obtaining the AG-ACNP certification exam. Once you have obtained your certification, we will discuss the sense of fulfillment you may experience as well as the plethora of new prospects that become available to you. In order to guarantee that you continue to offer the highest possible level of care to your patients, we will also go through ways to keep your certification current and continue to evolve as a practitioner.

The Path Forward: Professional Development and Advancement Opportunities

The need for AG-ACNPs is great, and there are several prospects for professional development and progress. Whether you choose to work in a hospital, an outpatient clinic, or a specialty unit, acute care nurse practitioners (AG-ACNPs) are in high demand because of their skill in the management of acute and complex medical diseases. An AG-ACNP has a dynamic career path that provides chances for specialization in fields such as cardiology, pulmonology, critical care, or emergency medicine. We will talk about the many different career paths that are open to you and give you advice on how to choose the one that is most compatible with your interests and ambitions.

The healthcare industry is in a state of constant change, and AG-ACNPs are in an excellent position to accommodate these alterations. In this lesson, we will investigate the developing tendencies and technologies that will shape the future of the healthcare industry. The landscape of patient care and the practice of nurse practitioners is undergoing significant change as a result of developments in telemedicine, artificial intelligence, and nursing informatics. By gaining an understanding of these advancements, you will be able to provide your patients with the most modern and beneficial care possible.

The Beginning of the Journey Is Now Before Us

As we embark on this trip into the realm of adult-gerontology acute care nursing and the road to certification, I want to encourage you to approach this journey with an open heart and a curious mind. It is more accurate to refer of nursing as a calling rather than a profession, particularly in the field of acute care. It's a promise to alleviate pain, promote health, and be a light of hope for individuals and their families when they need it the most.

This book is intended to be your constant companion, providing knowledge, direction, and support at every step of the way in whatever journey you may be on. If you are a student who is working hard to achieve your goals, a devoted nurse who is wanting to progress their career, or a healthcare professional who is enthusiastic about expanding their expertise, you will find important insights and practical resources within these pages. If you are a healthcare professional who is passionate about expanding their knowledge, you will also find useful insights and practical tools within these pages.

The examination to become an AG-ACNP is covered in Chapter 1.

The certification exam is the first step toward reaching the lofty goal of becoming an Adult-Gerontology Acute Care Nurse Practitioner (AG-ACNP). This remarkable accomplishment begins with the test. The exam required to earn the AG-ACNP certification is more than just a test; rather, it is the first step toward a rewarding career in the medical field. In this chapter, we will go deeply into the complexities of the certification test, including its purpose, format, substance, and the necessary methods to thrive on it.

The Importance of Receiving a Certification

Certification represents the completion of years of schooling, clinical experience, and a dedication to performing at a high level in the nursing profession. It indicates that you are prepared to provide advanced treatment to patients of any age, including adults and seniors, in acute care settings. However, it is much more than just a certificate; rather, it is a recognition of your passion to the profession and your commitment to provide treatment of the highest possible standard.

Why Obtaining Certification Is So Important

Recognition Receiving a certification defines you as an expert in your profession, elevating your status to one that is recognized and appreciated by both your colleagues and the employers who hire you as well as patients.

Patients are given the peace of mind that they will receive safe and effective care when they know that their caregivers are competent.

Opportunities for Progression in One's professional Acquiring a Certification makes one eligible for a greater variety of work openings and for professional progression.

Standardization: This ensures that all AG-ACNPs have the same degree of skill by establishing a standard for the practice of their profession.

Legal Requirements and Ethical Considerations The ability to practice as an AG-ACNP legally requires certification in several different jurisdictions.

Growth in One's field: Keeping one's certification current frequently necessitates continual education, which encourages continuous growth in one's field.

An Overview of the Certification Examination

Your knowledge, clinical abilities, and capacity to make good clinical decisions will all be evaluated thoroughly throughout the AG-ACNP certification exam. Its purpose is to evaluate whether or not you are prepared to work in acute care settings and handle the intricate health problems that are experienced by adult and geriatric patients.

Information Crucial to the Test

Eligibility: To be eligible, you normally need to be a licensed registered nurse (RN) with a Master's or Doctorate degree in nursing, and you also need to have completed the requisite coursework and clinical hours in an accredited AG-ACNP program. If you meet all of these requirements, then you are eligible.

The test is often administered on a computer and contains of questions with a variety of possible answers as well as clinical scenarios.

Time Restriction: In order to successfully finish the test, you will be given a predetermined amount of time, which will normally range from 3.5 to 4 hours.

The examination is based on the AG-ACNP test content outline, which is developed by either the American Nurses Credentialing Center (ANCC) or the American Association of Critical-Care Nurses (AACN), depending on the certifying body. Content: The exam is based on the AG-ACNP test content framework.

Score Required to Pass: The score required to pass can change, although it is often established at a level that corresponds to a baseline of knowledge in the subject area.

Outline of the Content of the Exam

The subject outline of the test will serve as your road map to success. It offers a comprehensive and granular description of the subjects and domains that will be tested throughout the examination. Take a look at the following example of a standard content outline:

The Cardiovascular System accounts for 20%

Problems with the heart

abnormalities of the vasculature

diseases related to hypertension

The Pulmonary System Accounts for 15%

Pulmonary conditions and illnesses

Failure of the respiratory system

Assistance with Ventilation

The Nervous System Comprises 15%

Evaluation of the nervous system

Disorders of the nervous system

Ischemic Attack

Ten percent is allocated to the digestive system.

Disorders of the gastrointestinal tract

Diseases of the liver and gallbladder

Renal and Urinary Systems Account for 10% of the Total

Disorders of the kidneys

Urinary system dysfunctions

Acute damage to the kidneys

Hematological and Immune Systems Account for 10% of the Total

Diseases of the blood and bone marrow

Immune system dysfunctions

Ten percent each goes to the professional role and the healthcare systems.

Models for the delivery of healthcare

Concerns of a moral and ethical nature

Policymaking and advocacy in the healthcare sector

Promotion of Health and Prevention of Diseases (5% of Total Cost)

Evaluation of the risks

Strategies for the promotion of health

Clinical Evaluation (5% of Total)

The processing and interpretation of data

The logic behind diagnosis

This content overview paints a detailed picture of the subjects on which you will be assessed as well as the relative importance of each of those subjects on the exam. Your preparation for the exam should be very similar to this outline, as this will ensure that you are well-prepared for both the breadth and the depth of the material.

Making Efforts to Prepare for the Test

The journey that is preparation for the AG-ACNP certification exam should not be underestimated. Acquiring knowledge, putting that knowledge to use in clinical settings, and becoming an expert in test-taking tactics are all necessary components. Let's get into the crucial actions that need to be taken in order to effectively prepare.

1. Construct a Learning Strategy

It is essential to design a study strategy that is well-organized. It assists you in allocating time to each content area, allowing you to ensure that you cover everything in a complete manner. Your strategy should take into account both your strong and weak points, allowing you to devote more of your attention to the more difficult aspects of the plan.

Define Exactly What You Want to Accomplish With Your Study Plan and Establish Precise Goals for Them. This can involve becoming an expert in certain content areas or reaching a certain score goal.

Determining how many hours of your week can be devoted to studying is the first step in time management. Make a schedule that you can follow because it is based on reality.

Break It Down: To make the subject overview more manageable, divide it up into chunks, and allot a certain amount of study time to each component. This helps to prevent cramming and ensures that all topics are covered thoroughly.

Evaluate Your Progress It is important to regularly examine your study strategy and to make any necessary revisions. If you are making good progress in one area, you can choose to devote more attention to an area that is performing less well.

Regular practice is important, and your study plan should include opportunities for you to evaluate both your level of comprehension and your ability to perform well on tests.

2. Collect the Required Study Materials

It is necessary to have the appropriate materials for research. For the purpose of assisting you in your preparation, you will require textbooks, online resources, practice exams, and clinical references.

Invest in comprehensive texts that cover the complete AG-ACNP scope of practice to ensure that you are prepared for the exam. These should be considered your primary source of information.

Explore the many online learning options, such as video lectures, online courses, and interactive study platforms, which are all available through internet resources.

Exam Practice: In order to get accustomed to the layout of the real exam and gauge your level of preparedness, you should take some mock exams. These might assist you in locating areas of weakness that require more attention.

References in Clinical Practice Be sure to always have references in clinical practice on available, since they are quite helpful when reviewing clinical guidelines and best practices.

3. Participate in some form of active learning.

Reading without participation is not enough on its own. Participate in active learning strategies to deepen your understanding and improve your ability to recall facts.

Participate in group studies by signing up for study groups or having conversations with other students. The act of explaining ideas to other people helps you to solidify your own comprehension.

Teach Back is when you teach the information to a learner in your head. This method compels you to have an understanding of the material that is good enough to describe it.

Clinical Application: If you are currently employed as a nurse, you should implement what you have learned into your daily clinical routine. Your theoretical understanding is strengthened by the practical experience you have gained here.

Self-Evaluation: On a regular basis, evaluate how well you comprehend the material by answering practice questions. This not only helps you retain information, but it also improves your ability to do well on tests.

4. Acquire Expertise in Test-Taking Techniques

It is not enough to simply know the material for the AG-ACNP certification exam; you must also demonstrate an understanding of how to approach the questions. The following is a list of helpful test-taking strategies:

Take Your Time and Read the Question: Pay close attention to the way that the question is posed. Try searching for words and phrases such as "most," "first," and "except." These words will direct your response.

Elimination Method: If you are unsure of the solution, utilize the method of elimination to eliminate options that are manifestly incorrect.

Regarding the management of your time, try not to spend an excessive amount of time on a single query. If you find yourself in a bind, it's best to walk on and come back to it later.

Mark for Review: If a question is difficult, you should mark it for review so that you can come back to it after you've answered questions that are simpler.

Follow your instincts: The first thing that comes to mind is frequently accurate. Try not to dwell on the past or second-guess your decisions.

Practice Under Realistic Test Conditions: When taking practice tests, you should simulate the conditions of the actual test. You will become more accustomed to the time pressure as a result of this.

Take Deep Breaths: If you want to manage your test anxiety, just keep cool and take deep breaths. Your performance may suffer if you're anxious, therefore it's important to learn how to relax.

Examine Your Responses If you have the opportunity and the time, examine your responses to ensure that you have not committed any sloppy errors.

5. Practice Exams and Detailed Feedback

It is quite beneficial to practice for actual tests. They provide a simulation of the actual testing environment and assist you in evaluating your level of preparedness. After you have completed a practice test, you should carefully check your answers, paying particular attention to the questions that you got wrong or were unclear about. Through the use of this technique, critical comments and valuable insights into areas that require improvement are obtained.

6. Seek Out Guidance and Support from Others

Do not be afraid to seek out to mentors, teachers, or experienced AG-ACNPs for advice and guidance if you are unsure about specific issues. They are able to offer elucidation as well as beneficial direction.

The Certification Exam is an Important Milestone in the Process

The AG-ACNP certification exam is more than just a test; it's a milestone in your route to becoming an expert in acute care nursing. The exam consists of multiple choice questions and a written component. It gives you the chance to show that you are dedicated to providing care that meets high standards, and it also paves the way for interesting new employment prospects.

The preparation for the exam is a multi-step process that needs commitment, the creation of a well-organized study plan, the identification of relevant resources, engaged learning, and an in-depth understanding of testing methodologies. As we progress through this book, we will discuss the fundamental clinical ideas and diagnostic reasoning abilities that will serve as the basis for your ability to perform well on the examination. You can confidently move on to the next step toward being a certified AG-ACNP if you put in the necessary amount of effort and take the appropriate strategy.

Keep in mind that obtaining certification is not the end goal of this trip; rather, it serves as a stepping stone on the path to a successful and satisfying profession. Your position as an AG-ACNP carries with it a significant amount of duty as well as privilege. You'll have the opportunity to make a major difference in the lives of adult and elderly patients at a time in their life when it matters the most. The information and abilities that you learn in preparation for the certification exam are not only for the purpose of passing the examination; rather, they are for delivering excellent care to those who are dependent on you.

Review of Fundamental Clinical Concepts is the Topic of Chapter 2.

In the realm of adult-gerontology acute care nursing, a profound and all-encompassing comprehension of fundamental clinical principles serves as the bedrock upon which efficient practice is constructed. This chapter delves into the critical clinical areas that an Adult-Gerontology Acute Care Nurse Practitioner (AG-ACNP) has to have under their belt in order to be successful. The cardiovascular system, the pulmonary system, the neurological system, the gastrointestinal system, the renal and urinary systems, the hematological and immunological systems, and other systems will all be covered in depth. These are the systems that you will most regularly come across in your profession, each of which will provide its own distinct set of challenges and factors to take into consideration.

The System of the Heart and Blood Vessels

It is common practice to refer to the cardiovascular system as the "lifeline" of the body. It is comprised of the heart, blood vessels, and blood, and its principal function is to remove waste items from the body while also ensuring that oxygen and nutrients are distributed evenly throughout the body. As an AG-ACNP, you will frequently come into contact with patients who are suffering from a variety of cardiovascular problems. It is essential to have a strong understanding of the anatomy and physiology of the cardiovascular system.

The Internal Structure of the Heart

The size of a closed fist, the heart is a muscular organ that is located in the chest between the lungs. It pumps blood throughout the body. It is composed of the following four chambers:

The right atrium is the location where blood that has been deoxygenated and returned from the body.

The right ventricle is responsible for pumping blood that has been deoxygenated to the lungs so that it can be oxygenated.

Left Atrium: This chamber is responsible for receiving oxygenated blood from the lungs.

The left ventricle is responsible for pumping oxygenated blood throughout the body via the circulatory system.

These chambers carry out their functions in a concerted manner so as to provide an uninterrupted blood flow. These four valves—the tricuspid, pulmonary, mitral (bicuspid), and aortic—are responsible for controlling the flow of blood through the heart by opening and closing at predetermined intervals.

Conditions of the Heart and Blood Vessels That Are Common

A accumulation of plaque in the coronary arteries, also known as coronary artery disease (CAD), which can result in chest pain (also known as angina) or a heart attack (also known as a myocardial infarction).

A condition known as congestive heart failure (CHF) occurs when the heart is unable to pump blood adequately, which causes fluid to build up in the lungs and the extremities.

Arrhythmias are a type of abnormal cardiac rhythm that can lead to symptoms such as palpitations, dizziness, and even fainting.

Diseases of the heart valves, including mitral regurgitation and aortic stenosis, are together referred to as valvular heart disease.

The medical term for high blood pressure is hypertension, and it is a major risk factor for cardiovascular illnesses.

Atherosclerosis in the peripheral arteries, most frequently in the legs, which results in decreased blood flow is referred to as peripheral artery disease (PAD).

Cardiomyopathy is a condition in which the heart muscle becomes weakened, limiting its capacity to adequately pump blood.

Important Clinical Evaluations to Consider

Comprehensive evaluations are absolutely necessary for people who suffer from cardiovascular conditions:

Cardiac auscultation involves listening to the sounds of the heart with a stethoscope. These sounds include the S1 (lub) and S2 (dub) sounds, as well as any murmurs, gallops, or additional heart sounds.

Measurement of Blood Pressure It is vitally important for people suffering from hypertension or any other cardiovascular condition to measure their blood pressure on a regular basis.

Electrocardiography (ECG) is a test that records the electrical activity of the heart and assists in the diagnosis of arrhythmias and other cardiac problems.

Echocardiography is a method of imaging that utilizes sound waves to make a moving image of the heart. This method is helpful in determining whether or not there are any abnormalities in the heart's valves.

Patients may choose to exercise or take medication in order to be subjected to a stress test in order to determine how their hearts react when subjected to increasing pressure.

Pharmacological Administration of Drugs

The study of cardiovascular pharmacology is an expansive field that includes the study of drugs that are used to treat a variety of ailments. The following are some examples of common drug classes:

Beta-blockers are medications that slow the heart rate and lower blood pressure. They are frequently prescribed for the treatment of hypertension and irregular heart rhythms.

Inhibitors of the enzyme angiotensin-converting enzyme (ACE) are a class of medications that assist relax blood arteries and reduce blood pressure.

Diuretics are a type of medication that is frequently prescribed to people who suffer from heart failure.

Antiplatelet Agents: Medications such as aspirin prevent platelets from aggregating into clots by minimizing the potential for clot formation.

Statins are medications that bring cholesterol levels down and cut down on the likelihood of developing atherosclerosis.

Anticoagulants are medications that are provided to patients to prevent the formation of blood clots. Examples of these medications include warfarin and newer medicines such as apixaban.

Considerations Regarding Cardiovascular Health When Aging

Patients who are elderly frequently have special cardiovascular issues to take into account:

The heart naturally goes through a process of structural and functional change as we age, which results in a decrease in the heart's overall efficiency.

Frailty is a condition that can affect older persons and can make them more susceptible to the effects of cardiovascular stresses.

Polypharmacy refers to the practice of geriatric individuals taking numerous drugs, which raises the possibility of adverse reactions and drug interactions.

Comorbidity: In patients over the age of 65, cardiovascular disease is frequently accompanied by other chronic illnesses, such as diabetes or hypertension.

In order to provide appropriate care to elderly patients who suffer from cardiovascular diseases, it is essential to have a solid understanding of these age-specific characteristics.

The Lungs and the Pulmonary System

Another crucial component of your profession is the pulmonary system, which is in charge of eliminating carbon dioxide from the blood and delivering oxygen to the bloodstream. It is especially important to keep this in mind when working in acute care settings, where you can come into contact with patients who are experiencing respiratory distress or acute pulmonary diseases.

The Structure and Function of the Respiratory System

The trachea, the bronchi, and the bronchioles make up the airways that are a part of the respiratory system. The lungs and the muscles that control breathing are also a part of this system. Alveoli are the microscopic air sacs in which the process of gas exchange takes place. During the process of exhalation, oxygen is delivered to the bloodstream, while carbon dioxide is eliminated from the body.

Conditions of the Lungs That Are Common

Pneumonia is an illness that affects the lung tissue and is frequently accompanied by symptoms such as coughing, fever, and difficulty breathing.

COPD stands for chronic obstructive pulmonary disease and refers to a group of lung disorders that are characterized by a restriction of airflow. These diseases include chronic bronchitis and emphysema.

A chronic disorder that causes inflammation of the airways, which in turn leads to repeated wheezing and shortness of breath is known as asthma.

A pulmonary embolism, often known as a PE, is a blood clot that plugs a pulmonary artery, resulting in sudden chest pain and trouble breathing.

Acute Respiratory Distress Syndrome (ARDS) is a severe lung illness that is characterized by significant oxygen deficit and is typically found in critically ill individuals.

Pulmonary hypertension is a condition in which the arteries of the lungs have high blood pressure, resulting in symptoms such as shortness of breath and chest pain.

Important Clinical Evaluations to Consider

The auscultation of the lungs is an extremely important diagnostic tool. Crackling, wheezing, and a general quieting of the breather are all signs that there may be underlying problems.

An x-ray of the chest, often known as a chest radiograph, can produce images of the lungs and point out abnormalities such as infiltrates in pneumonia.

Pulmonary function tests, often known as PFTs, evaluate a patient's lung capacity and are helpful in the diagnostic process for illnesses such as asthma and COPD.

Arterial Blood Gases (ABGs) are vital for determining how to treat respiratory distress because they measure the amounts of oxygen and carbon dioxide in the blood.

Invasive process known as bronchoscopy, which allows for visualization of the airways as well as the collection of samples for diagnostic analysis.

Pharmacological Administration of Drugs

The treatment of pulmonary problems typically entails the use of a wide variety of drugs, including:

Bronchodilators are drugs that relax the muscles in the airways, which leads to an increase in airflow. Ipratropium and albuterol are two examples of such medications.

Inhaled corticosteroids are a typical treatment for asthma and chronic obstructive pulmonary disease (COPD) because they reduce inflammation in the airways.

Antibiotics are absolutely necessary for the treatment of bacterial infections such as pneumonia.

Anticoagulants are medications that are used to treat cases of pulmonary embolism by preventing the formation of further blood clots.

Pulmonary vasodilators are medications that relax the blood arteries in the lungs and are used to treat pulmonary hypertension.

Considerations Regarding the Lungs in Gerontology

Alterations in a person's respiratory system that occur naturally with aging can have an effect on their lung function. There is a possibility that you will work with elderly patients who suffer from conditions such as diminished lung compliance or decreased respiratory muscle strength. Alterations in the immune system that come with getting older might also increase the likelihood of getting a respiratory infection.

The Nervous and Nervous System

When it comes to the proper operation of the body as a whole, the neurological system is absolutely essential. Your knowledge of neurological assessment and fundamental principles is extremely helpful due to the fact that acute neurological problems are frequently seen in the course of AG-ACNP practice.

The Structure and Function of the Nervous System

The brain and the spinal cord are the two primary components of the nervous system.

The Central Nervous System (CNS) is comprised of both the brain and the spinal cord, and it is responsible for controlling the majority of the body's processes.

The Peripheral Nervous System, often known as the PNS, is the part of the nervous system that is located outside of the Central Nervous System (CNS).

The central nervous system (CNS) is in charge of controlling vital activities like as consciousness, movement, and coordination. The PNS acts as a communication bridge between the central nervous system (CNS) and the rest of the body, so enabling both sensory input and muscular output.

Disorders of the Nervous System That Are Common

A stroke is an occurrence that can occur in the cerebrovascular system when there is a disturbance in the blood flow to the brain. This can result in sudden neurological impairments.

Seizures are characterized by uncontrolled electrical activity in the brain, which can present in a number of different ways.

Trauma to the Head and Brain: Head and brain injuries can range from mild concussions to severe traumatic brain injuries (TBIs), and everything in between.

Infections of the Nervous System Neurological symptoms can be caused by a variety of conditions, including meningitis and encephalitis.

Neurodegenerative disorders include Alzheimer's disease and Parkinson's disease, both of which can lead to a gradual loss in brain function.

Neuromuscular Disorders include myasthenia gravis and amyotrophic lateral sclerosis (ALS), both of which are diseases that affect the nerves and muscles in the body.

Important Clinical Evaluations to Consider

An evaluation of the patient's mental condition, cranial nerves, motor function, sensory function, coordination, and reflexes are all part of the neurological examination.

Imaging: computed tomography (CT) and magnetic resonance imaging (MRI) scans are frequently used to image the brain and discover abnormalities.

The electroencephalogram, sometimes known as an EEG, is a vital tool for detecting seizure disorders because it records the electrical activity in the brain.

The invasive operation known as a lumbar puncture is performed to collect cerebrospinal fluid, which is helpful for identifying neurological illnesses.

Evaluation of muscle strength and function, typically accomplished through the use of electromyography (EMG). Also known as a neuromuscular assessment.

Pharmacological Administration of Drugs

When providing therapy for neurological conditions, there is a wide range of options available for drugs to choose from. The following are some examples:

Tissue Plasminogen Activator, or tPA, is a drug that is administered to patients suffering from acute strokes in order to break up blood clots and restore blood flow to the brain.

Antiepileptic Drugs are medicines such as phenytoin and levetiracetam that are used to treat and prevent seizures.

Analgesics are commonly prescribed for the treatment of pain associated with illnesses such as migraines and neuropathic pain.

Disease-Modifying Agents are drugs like donepezil and levodopa, which are used to treat Alzheimer's and Parkinson's, respectively.

Relaxants for the muscles are helpful in treating disorders that cause muscular spasms or spasticity.

Considerations of the Brain's Aging Process in Gerontology

It is possible to come across age-related neurological illnesses in the elderly population, such as cognitive decline or neurodegenerative disorders. Your capacity to give care that is focused on the needs of the patient is even more essential when dealing with elderly patients who frequently demand specific attention, particularly in instances of delirium or dementia.

The Digestive and Pancreatic Systems

The digestive process and the uptake of nutrients are both greatly influenced by the gastrointestinal (GI) system. It is absolutely necessary to have a fundamental understanding of the GI in order to diagnose and treat acute and chronic GI problems.

Anatomy of the Gastrointestinal System

The digestive system includes not only the mouth and the esophagus but also the stomach, the small intestine, and the large intestine. The process of digestion starts in the mouth, where food is first chewed and then crushed into smaller pieces before being transported down the esophagus and into the stomach. The majority of nutritional absorption takes place in the small intestine, whereas the large intestine is responsible for the digestion of food, the absorption of water, and the creation of feces.

The Most Frequent GI Ailments

Heartburn and regurgitation are symptoms of a disorder known as gastroesophageal reflux disease (GERD), which occurs when acid from the stomach rushes backward into the esophagus.

Peptic ulcers are wounds that form in the lining of the stomach or the first section of the small intestine and are frequently brought on by H. pylori. microorganisms known as pylori.

Inflammatory Bowel Disease, abbreviated as IBD, is an umbrella name comprising illnesses such as Crohn's disease and ulcerative colitis, both of which are characterized by persistent inflammation of the digestive tract.

The inflammation of the intestines and stomach is known as gastroenteritis and is most commonly caused by infections with viruses or bacteria.

Inflammation or infection of the tiny pouches that can occur in the walls of the colon; this condition is known as diverticulitis.

Hepatitis is an inflammation of the liver, which is most commonly caused by infections caused by viruses.

Important Clinical Evaluations to Consider

During the abdominal examination, the physician will palpate the patient's belly and check for pain as well as lumps.

Endoscopy is a potentially invasive treatment that allows for visualization of the gastrointestinal tract and, if necessary, the collection of biopsies.

Stool analysis is helpful for determining how well the digestive system is working and locating problems such as malabsorption.

Tests of liver function evaluate the organ's capacity to digest the numerous chemicals that are present in the blood.

A colonoscopy is an examination of the large intestine, and it is a vital diagnostic tool for the diagnosis of colon cancer as well as other conditions.

Pharmacological Administration of Drugs

Intestinal and digestive disorders are frequently treated with a wide variety of pharmaceuticals, including:

In disorders such as gastroesophageal reflux disease (GERD), proton pump inhibitors (PPIs) are taken to lower the amount of acid produced by the stomach.

Antibiotics are medications that are recommended for infections such as H. pylori in those who have peptic ulcers.

Anti-inflammatory drugs are frequently used in the treatment of inflammatory bowel disease (IBD).

Antiemetics are a class of medications used to treat and prevent nausea and vomiting.

Laxatives are medications that are taken in cases of constipation to stimulate bowel movements.

Gerontology Taking into Account GI Considerations

Changes that occur as a result of aging can have an effect on the function of the gastrointestinal (GI) system. For example, decreased production of stomach acid might have an impact on the ability to absorb nutrients. You also run the risk of developing gastrointestinal disorders that are more common in people of advanced age, such as diverticulosis.

Systems of the Kidneys and Urinary Bladder

A healthy fluid and electrolyte balance, as well as the elimination of waste products from the body, are dependent on the function of the kidneys and the urinary system. These systems are essential for the management of both acute and chronic diseases, including acute kidney injury (AKI) and chronic kidney disease (CKD), which are abbreviated respectively.

The structure and function of the renal system

The two kidneys that make up the renal system are responsible for filtering the blood in order to remove waste and excess substances, ultimately leading to the formation of urine. Urine leaves the kidneys and passes via the ureters on its way to the bladder. The bladder is where urine is stored until being expelled through the urethra.

Common disorders of the kidneys and urinary tract

Acute kidney injury (AKI) refers to a sudden loss of kidney function, which is typically brought on by situations such as dehydration or the toxicity of certain medications.

Chronic Kidney Disease (CKD) refers to a gradual and ongoing loss of kidney function that, if left untreated, can eventually result in end-stage renal disease (ESRD).

Urinary tract infections, sometimes known as UTIs, are infections that can either damage the bladder (a condition known as cystitis) or the kidneys (a condition known as pyelonephritis).

Nephrolithiasis refers to the production of kidney stones, which can result in excruciating discomfort and an obstruction of the urinary tract.

Glomerulonephritis is an inflammation of the glomeruli, which are the units in the kidneys that are responsible for filtering blood.

Renal hypertension is a form of high blood pressure that is caused by issues with the kidneys and is frequently related with chronic kidney disease (CKD).

Important Clinical Evaluations to Consider

Urinalysis is the process of examining the patient's urine to look for abnormalities such as blood, protein, or indications of illness.

These two blood tests are used to evaluate kidney function: serum creatinine and blood urea nitrogen, also known as BUN.

Imaging of the kidneys using ultrasound technology to determine their size, shape, and whether or not they have any abnormalities.

CT scans and MRIs are helpful diagnostic tools for identifying kidney stones and other structural problems.

A biopsy of the kidney is an invasive procedure that is performed to acquire tissue samples for diagnostic purposes.

Pharmacological Administration of Drugs

Medications that are used to treat infections, manage pain, or control blood pressure are frequently a part of the renal and urinary disease care process. In the event that ESRD is present, it is possible that renal replacement therapies such as hemodialysis or peritoneal dialysis will be required.

Gerontological Aspects Regarding the Kidneys

Patients of advanced age are at increased risk of developing age-related changes in their kidney function, which can result in a diminished capacity to filter and eliminate waste products. Conditions affecting the kidneys can become more difficult to manage in older people, so you should be ready to handle the specific requirements of these patients.

The Systems of the Blood and the Immune Response

The hematological system, which is comprised of the blood and the organs that create blood, is an essential component in the processes of oxygen transportation, blood coagulation, and immunological defense. As an AG-ACNP, you will frequently come into contact with patients who are suffering from a wide variety of hematological and immunological diseases.

The Structure and Function of the Hematological System

The blood, the bone marrow, and the lymphatic system are all components of the hematological system. Platelets (thrombocytes), white blood cells (leukocytes), and red blood cells (erythrocytes) are the three components that make up blood. Lymph nodes, the spleen, and lymphatic veins are all components of the lymphatic system, which is responsible for maintaining immunological function.

Conditions Related to the Immune System and the Blood

Anemia is a disorder that is characterized by a decreased red blood cell count or decreased hemoglobin levels, both of which can lead to feelings of exhaustion and weakness.

Thrombocytopenia is a decrease in the number of platelets in the blood, which can lead to increased risk of bleeding and bruising.

Cancer of the bone marrow and blood, often known as leukemia, which results in abnormal production of white blood cells.

Lymphoma is a form of cancer that affects the lymphatic system. The most frequent varieties of lymphoma are Hodgkin's and non-Hodgkin's lymphomas.

Hemophilia is a genetic condition that makes it difficult for the blood to clot.

Autoimmune disorders include conditions such as rheumatoid arthritis, multiple sclerosis, and systemic lupus erythematosus (SLE).

Immunodeficiency disorders are conditions in which the immune system is weakened, making the patient more susceptible to infections.

Important Clinical Evaluations to Consider

A complete blood count, often known as a CBC, is a test that measures the number of red blood cells, white blood cells, and platelets in the patient's blood.

The coagulation profile evaluates the function of blood clotting, which is essential for diagnosing and treating diseases such as hemophilia.

Aspiration and biopsy of the bone marrow are invasive procedures that are used to investigate bone marrow cells for a variety of diseases.

An examination of the lymph nodes involves palpation and evaluation of the nodes to determine whether or not they are painful or enlarged.

Tests of Immune Function Measure the functionality of the immune system and discover any inadequacies.

Pharmacological Administration of Drugs

To effectively treat hematological and immunological problems, medication is frequently required. These treatments may be used to stimulate the formation of blood cells, reduce inflammation, or treat autoimmune diseases. Clotting factor replacement therapy could be required for patients who have bleeding issues that are particularly severe.

In the field of gerontology, hematological considerations are essential.

Hematological changes in older persons can include a reduction in the activity of the bone marrow, which can contribute to the development of anemia. Aging can also cause a reduction in immune function, which can make elderly individuals more prone to catching illnesses.

Advanced Clinical Assessment is the topic of Chapter 3.

The advanced clinical evaluation serves as the cornerstone upon which the excellence of the adult-geriatric acute care nursing practice is built. This chapter digs into the complexities of clinical evaluation and places an emphasis on the vital role that it plays in patient care, diagnosis, and the planning of therapy. It is crucial for you, as an Adult-Gerontology Acute treatment Nurse Practitioner (AG-ACNP), to be able to undertake advanced clinical assessments so that you can provide comprehensive treatment that is based on evidence to adult and geriatric patients who are receiving care in acute care settings.

The Importance of Performing Clinical Evaluations

The clinical evaluation is the foundation of the healthcare system. It is a methodical procedure that involves acquiring and analyzing information on patients so that decisions about their health can be made in an informed manner. The AG-ACNP places a significant emphasis on clinical assessment in order to:

Establish a Baseline: Determine the patient's current state of health and evaluate it in comparison to the data from the baseline.

Conditions are identified during the diagnostic process, which can include both acute and chronic disorders.

Assess the patient's response to the treatment and treatments being administered while monitoring their progress.

Adjust Interventions: Care plans should be adapted to the specific requirements of each individual patient.

To achieve better patient outcomes, care must be provided in a timely and suitable manner in order to boost the patient's overall health.

The Combined Craft and Science of Clinical Evaluation

Assessment in the clinical setting combines elements of both art and science. The ability to communicate with patients, empathy, and the capacity to build relationships with them are all essential components of the "art" part of medicine, which is responsible for the efficient collection of information. The "science" component entails the methodical gathering of data, analysis of those findings, critical thinking, and the making of therapeutic decisions. A comprehensive method of treating patients is produced as a result of the confluence of these different aspects.

Components of a More Advanced Clinical Assessment

The advanced clinical evaluation is comprised of numerous essential components, each of which contributes to an in-depth comprehension of the health of the patient. These parts include the following:

Collecting a comprehensive medical history that includes current symptoms, historical medical issues, family history, and social history is part of the process known as "health history." The subsequent evaluation will be based on the basis laid by this material.

The patient's body is subjected to a methodical inspection, as well as palpation, percussion, and auscultation as part of the physical examination. It gives incredibly helpful information regarding the patient's physical status, including vital signs, appearance, and organ systems.

Ordering and interpreting laboratory tests, radiographic examinations, and other diagnostic procedures in order to confirm or rule out certain disorders is referred to as diagnostic testing.

An evaluation of the patient's mental health, emotional well-being, and their capacity to carry out activities of daily living (ADLs) is included in the assessment of their psychosocial and functional status. Geriatric individuals absolutely require an evaluation of both their social support and their functional state.

Conducting tailored examinations based on the patient's major complaint or specific ailment, frequently includes a careful examination of the affected area. This type of assessment is referred to as "focused assessment."

The study of medical history serves as the basis for evaluation.

The medical history of the patient is an important source of data since it reveals information about the patient's present health status, as well as any previous medical disorders and relevant risk factors. A complete medical history will include the following:

1. Currently Existing Illness

The primary complaint is the primary cause for seeking medical attention.

The history of the present sickness is a comprehensive narrative of the current health problems, including the onset, progression, accompanying symptoms, and variables that either alleviate or exacerbate the problem.

2. Previous conditions and treatments

Documenting all previous medical diagnoses and ongoing illnesses requires careful attention to detail.

Surgical history includes listing all procedures, along with the dates for each one and the results.

Documenting current and previous medications, including over-the-counter and herbal supplements, is an important part of medication management.

Identifying pharmacological, food, or environmental allergies and reactions is part of the process of dealing with allergies.

Reviewing the patient's vaccination history is part of the immunization process.

3. The past of the family

Keeping a record of the medical illnesses that affect members of a family, particularly those that may have a hereditary component, such as diabetes, cancer, or heart disease.

4. The history of society

Assessing one's usage of cigarettes, alcohol, and other substances is one of the lifestyle factors.

Understanding the patient's work environment and identifying any potential hazards to the patient's occupational health is essential.

Examining the patient's living conditions and support network is part of the living situation assessment.

The gathering of information regarding sexual activities, partnerships, and hazards is referred to as sexual history.

Recognizing cultural ideas, behaviors, and traditions that may have an effect on healthcare decisions is referred to as "cultural factors."

5. An Examination of the Systems

A thorough examination of each body system, during which the patient is questioned about any symptoms or problems that they may be experiencing, regardless of whether or not they appear to be directly related to the patient's primary complaint.

6. Evaluation of Functionality

Activities of Daily Living, often known as ADLs, are an evaluation of a patient's capacity to carry out fundamental acts of self-care, such as taking a shower, getting dressed, and eating.

Activities of Daily Living Instrumental (ADL Instrumental): Evaluating more complicated tasks such as handling funds, preparing meals, and arranging transportation.

Evaluation of a person's cognitive function involves testing their memory, thinking, and ability to solve problems.

7. Evaluation of Psychosocial Factors

Asking about a person's mood, feelings, and whether they are experiencing any symptoms of anxiety or depression is part of maintaining good mental health.

The process of determining the causes of stress, which may include problems in the family, worries about money, or recent changes in one's life.

The Hands-On Approach Is Taken in the Physical Examination

The patient is subjected to a series of inspections, palpations, percussions, and auscultations as part of the physical examination, which is a hands-on, methodical process. Its purpose is to detect problems in the physical structure, evaluate organ systems, and collect essential data. A comprehensive exam should cover the following areas, even if the scope of the physical examination can change based on the patient's condition and the primary complaint that they have.

1. Aspects Relating to the Whole

Examination of the patient's general appearance, including the presence or absence of symptoms of distress, posture, and general disposition.

Assessment of vital signs includes taking temperature, blood pressure, heart rate, and respiration rate, as well as measuring oxygen saturation.

2. Examination of the Head and Neck

Examination of the head, including the hair and the face.

Visual acuity, pupillary response, and fundoscopy are all components of the eye exam that will be performed.

examination of the ears, including testing of hearing as well as looking for any signs of discharge or irritation.

Examining the nose and searching for any signs of congestion, discharge, or abnormalities are all important parts of this step.

Examining the oral cavity, including the mouth, gums, teeth, and throat, as well as looking for any abnormalities.

3. Examination of the Heart and Blood Vessels

chest palpation and evaluation of movement of the chest wall should be performed.

Percussion to evaluate the dullness of the heart rhythm.

Evaluation of the patient's heart rate and rhythm, as well as auscultation of the heart's noises.

Examination of the patient's peripheral pulses, including evaluation of their strength and symmetry via palpation.

4. Examination of the Respiratory System

Examination of the chest to look for any abnormalities or differences in shape.

A feeling of fullness and tenderness in the chest is palpated.

Utilization of percussion in order to evaluate lung resonance.

Auscultation of the sounds of the patient's breath, listening for wheezing, crackling, or any other irregularities.

5. An Examination of the Abdomen

Examining the abdomen for any distension, scars, or lumps that may be present.

Listening for sounds coming from the gut.

Palpation is done to determine how delicate an organ is and its size.

Utilization of percussive techniques in order to identify organ boundaries and fluid accumulations.

6. Examination of the Nervous System

evaluation of the patient's mental health, including assessment of orientation and responsiveness.

evaluation of the cranial nerves, including tests of vision, eye movements, facial sensibility, and hearing.

An analysis of the patient's motor and sensory function.

Examination of reflexes, including plantar and deep tendon reflexes, as well as other reflexes.

7. Examination of the Musculoskeletal System

Examination to look for deformities, edema, or anomalies in the joints.

assessment of muscle strength as well as discomfort when palpating the area.

Joints are tested for their range of motion.

8. An Examination of the Skin and Extremities

Conduct a thorough examination, looking for rashes, lesions, and other signs of trauma.

Evaluation of the color and warmth of the skin.

An evaluation of the patient's limbs to check for cyanosis, clubbing, and edema.

9. Examination of the Genitourinary Tract

Evaluation of the structures of the vaginal and urinary systems, including the search for any masses or anomalies that may be present.

Evaluation of urine elimination to determine frequency, urgency, and dysuria in addition to other symptoms.

10. Additional Analysis of the Specifics of the System

examinations that are customized to the patient's primary symptom or condition, such as a focused neurological examination for a patient who is complaining of headaches or a musculoskeletal examination for a patient who is complaining of joint pain.

Testing for Diagnostic Purposes: Going Beyond the Physical Exam

In most instances, diagnostic testing is included as part of the comprehensive assessment in addition to the physical examination that is performed. These tests provide objective data that can be used to confirm or rule out certain illnesses, track the progression of disease, or evaluate how effectively a treatment is working. The following are some examples of diagnostic tests:

1. Laboratory Examinations

The complete blood count (CBC), the comprehensive metabolic panel (CMP), and the lipid profile are all examples of blood tests that measure the levels of a variety of chemicals.

Examinations to determine the state of an organ's functionality may include things like liver function tests and renal function examinations.

investigations of coagulation, including the prothrombin time (PT), the activated partial thromboplastin time (aPTT), and the international normalized ratio (INR).

levels of hormones, as well as tests to evaluate thyroid function.

a battery of microbiological testing, including viral load assays and blood cultures.

2. Investigations Using Radiation

X-rays are used to see the tissues and bones.

CT scans, which stand for computed tomography, are used to provide detailed images of cross sections.

Magnetic resonance imaging, sometimes known as MRI, is a technique used to get high-resolution images of soft tissues.

Utilization of ultrasound to examine blood flow and inside organs.

Scans performed in nuclear medicine for the purpose of functionally imaging organs and tissues.

PET scans, which stand for positron emission tomography, are used to investigate metabolic activities within the body.

3. Examination of the Heart

Electrocardiography, sometimes known as an ECG or EKG, is a recording of the electrical activity of the heart.

The use of echocardiography to obtain a visual of the structure and function of the heart.

Evaluation of the patient's heart function under a variety of stressful settings may involve stress tests, such as those using exercise or pharmaceutical agents.

4. Examination of Your Lung Function

Spirometry is used to evaluate lung function by measuring things like lung volumes and airflow.

Analysis of the arterial blood gas (ABG) to determine the concentrations of oxygen and carbon dioxide in the blood.

5. Endoscopy as well as Biopsies

Endoscopic examinations of the gastrointestinal tract, including upper endoscopy and colonoscopy.

Bronchoscopy is performed in order to examine the airways and collect samples.

Biopsies of the affected tissue to analyze the cellular changes and provide a diagnosis of illnesses such as cancer.

6. Diagnostic Imaging and Therapeutic Interventions

Angiography is used to view blood arteries and evaluate how much blood is flowing through them.

Interventions performed with a catheter, such as angioplasty and the implantation of stents.

Procedures for taking biopsies that are image-guided.

7. Examination at the Molecular and Genetic Levels

PCR, which stands for polymerase chain reaction, and sequencing of DNA are used to find genetic alterations.

Molecular markers to direct focused therapy for particular illnesses, such as cancer.

Evaluation of the Psychosocial and Functional State

Assessing a patient's mental health as well as their physical and mental capabilities is an essential component of patient care, particularly when working with adult and elderly patients. The patient's psychological well-being as well as their functional capacities have a significant impact on both their overall health and their reaction to treatment.

Evaluation of Psychosocial Factors

Inquire about the patient's mental health, including their mood, feelings, and whether or not they are exhibiting any symptoms of anxiety, sadness, or any other psychiatric illnesses.

Identifying the patient's stressors is important since these factors have the potential to have a major effect on the patient's health. Concerns about one's family, one's finances, one's place of employment, or even just recent life changes can all be sources of stress.

System of Support It is important to evaluate the patient's social support system, which should include family, friends, and resources from the community. In order to effectively deal with one's disease and make a full recovery, having supportive relationships is essential.

Recognize the patient's cultural ideas, customs, and traditions in order to account for cultural factors. When it comes to providing patient-centered care and resolving cultural inequities in healthcare, having cultural competence is absolutely necessary.

Evaluation of Functionality

The patient's capacity to carry out routine tasks and continue living independently are the primary areas of focus during a functional assessment. The following are two major aspects of the functional assessment:

The term "activities of daily living," or "ADLs," refers to the fundamental acts of self-care that are required for daily life. They consist of things like taking a shower, getting dressed, grooming oneself, eating, and going to the bathroom. When trying to measure a patient's level of independence, it is helpful to evaluate their capacity to execute ADLs.

IADL stands for instrumental activities of daily living, which refer to activities that are more difficult and call on both mental and physical capabilities. Taking care of one's money, preparing meals, going shopping, maintaining one's home, and driving oneself to and from work are some examples. The patient's functional independence and their capacity to live independently in the community can be gleaned from the evaluation of their IADLs.

Functional evaluations are of utmost significance for geriatric patients since they assist in the identification of age-related changes in function as well as possible areas that could benefit from support or intervention. Impairments in activities of daily living and instrumental activities of daily living can be an indicator of the need for additional care or services, such as assistance with home health or assisted living.

Assessment That Is Concentrated and Tailored to the Primary Concern

When a patient appears at an acute care facility with a particular disease or chief complaint, it is often required to perform a targeted assessment on the patient. The scope of this particular type of evaluation is narrowed in order to collect pertinent data in relation to the patient's primary health concern. The following are components of a focused assessment:

Obtaining a Detailed History involves inquiring about particular aspects of the patient's primary complaint, such as the origin and course of symptoms, connected causes, and any past occurrences, through the use of specific inquiries.

Performing a Targeted Physical Examination involves putting more of an emphasis on the examination of the damaged area or system, with a particular focus on the signs and symptoms that are relevant.

The second step in the diagnostic process is called "ordering diagnostic tests," and it involves selecting the proper tests or studies that can provide additional information about the illness. These may include imaging investigations, laboratory testing, or specialized evaluations.

The AG-ACNP is able to quickly acquire essential data thanks to the focused assessment, which then enables them to make educated decisions regarding diagnosis, treatment, and care planning. It is an effective method for coping with acute illnesses and providing direction for interventions.

Evaluation of Patients in Their Golden Years

When evaluating elderly patients, it is necessary to take into account a number of specific factors due to the distinctive characteristics of this demographic. Patients in their geriatric years frequently arrive with several chronic diseases, changes associated with aging, and intricate psychosocial requirements. During the evaluation of elderly patients, it is important to keep in mind the following factors:

A comprehensive geriatric assessment, often known as a CGA, is a multidimensional evaluation that analyzes the physical, functional, mental, and social aspects of the health of older patients. The CGA assists in the identification of vulnerabilities and the development of individualized care plans.

Polypharmacy is the practice of a patient taking many drugs, which increases the potential for harmful effects and drug interactions. Geriatric individuals typically engage in this practice. It is vital to conduct a comprehensive examination of the medications.

Assess the patient for geriatric syndromes such as frailty, cognitive impairment, falls, and incontinence. These conditions are frequent in the elderly and can have an effect on their general health and well-being.

Cultural Competence: Show sensitivity to different cultures and be knowledgeable about the wide range of experiences and beliefs held by geriatric patients. It is impossible to provide treatment that is centered on the patient without cultural competence.

During the process of advance care planning, the patient's wishes about end-of-life care and advance directives should be discussed and documented. The process of making decisions for one's end-of-life care is an essential part of geriatric care.

Assessing the patient's functional status should center on determining whether or not they are able to carry out activities of daily living and instrumental activities of daily living. Determine the impairments that could benefit from support or interventions.

Assess the patient's cognitive function and look for signs of cognitive abnormalities such as dementia in the cognitive assessment. A prompt diagnosis enables appropriate interventions and assistance to be provided.

Assessing the Patient's Fall Risk It is important to assess the patient's risk of falling, as this is a common cause for concern among the elderly population. When it's appropriate, put fall prevention methods into action.

Keeping records and producing documentation

One essential component of advanced clinical assessment is the creation of documentation that is both accurate and exhaustive. To guarantee that all assessment data, findings, diagnostic results, and interventions are recorded and can be accessed by the healthcare team, proper documentation must be completed. The documentation serves multiple objectives, including the following:

Communication: It makes it possible for healthcare personnel to communicate effectively with one another, which ensures that all members of the team are kept abreast of the patient's condition and requirements.

Legal Protection Complete documentation can be used as a legal record of the care that was delivered, safeguarding healthcare practitioners from liability in the event that a legal issue arises.

Care Continuity: Care continuity is promoted by thorough documentation since it enables different providers to pick up where others have left off, so guaranteeing a smooth transfer from one to the next.

Quality Improvement: It contributes to quality improvement by supplying data for analysis and evaluation of care procedures and outcomes, which in turn helps support efforts to enhance quality.

Information on patients that has been meticulously documented is invaluable for the purposes of research and education as well as for the planning of healthcare.

The following components should be included in any good documentation:

Detailed account of one's medical history, including current and former illnesses, treatments, and allergic reactions.

a comprehensive report of the findings of the physical examination, including an analysis of vital signs and organ systems.

The findings of diagnostic tests and how they should be interpreted.

An examination that is concentrated on the patient's primary ailment or complaint in particular.

Assessment of the patient's psychosocial circumstances, including their mental health, sources of stress, support networks, and cultural factors.

Evaluation of functionality, with a focus on elderly people in particular.

Details concerning desires for future medical care and care at the end of life.

Medication lists that are both accurate and up to date.

Plans of care, which may include a diagnosis, strategies for treatment, and desired outcomes.

Notes on the patient's progress that capture any changes in their condition and how they have responded to any interventions.

Consent given after being fully educated about a medical procedure or therapy.

The patient's level of comprehension of the information, as well as any patient education that was provided.

The documentation needs to be understandable, succinct, and compliant with the standards of the company as well as the legal requirements. Electronic health record (EHR) systems are routinely utilized for documentation, and practitioners of healthcare should obtain training on these systems to ensure that record keeping is accurate and efficient.

The Diagnostic Reasoning Approach, Chapter 4

It is essential for Adult-Gerontology Acute Care Nurse Practitioners (AG-ACNPs) to have strong diagnostic reasoning skills in order to be successful in clinical practice. This chapter delves into the fundamental aspects of diagnostic reasoning, the process of clinical reasoning, and many methods that can help you improve your diagnostic abilities. It is essential for you, as an AG-ACNP, to be able to make diagnoses that are both accurate and prompt if you want to improve patient outcomes in acute care settings.

The Importance of Using a Diagnosis to Guide Treatment

Diagnostic reasoning refers to the process that medical professionals go through to collect, examine, and interpret a patient's clinical data in order to ascertain the patient's current state of health and identify any issues that are associated with their physical wellbeing. It is a talent that encompasses a wide range of responsibilities and helps bridge the gap between diagnosis and therapy. An accurate diagnosis serves as the foundation for making decisions on treatment, which in turn ensures that patients receive the necessary attention. The following is why diagnostic reasoning is so important:

Care Focused on the Patient An accurate diagnosis makes it possible to develop individualized treatment programs that are patient-centered and that are designed to meet the specific requirements and conditions of each individual patient.

Treatment Planning: The diagnosis serves as a guide in selecting the most appropriate treatments, interventions, and therapies, which in turn improves the efficacy of care.

Patient Safety: An accurate diagnosis lowers the likelihood of medication errors, adverse events, and unnecessary treatments, which all contribute to an increased level of patient safety.

Allocation of Resources: Making an accurate diagnosis assists in effectively allocating available resources, which in turn ensures that patients receive the appropriate amount of treatment.

Preventative Measures: An early and accurate diagnosis makes it possible to take preventative measures, which may arrest the progression of diseases or consequences.

The Deductive Thinking Behind the Diagnosis

The diagnostic reasoning process is comprised of a number of processes that are carried out in sequential order in order for medical professionals to arrive at a diagnosis. As a reflection of the changing nature of clinical practice, these processes are iterative and frequently overlap with one another. The following is an outline of the diagnostic reasoning process:

Data Collection: The first step in the process is to collect data by doing a medical history review, a physical examination, laboratory testing, and any other diagnostic examinations that may be necessary. In this phase, you will collect useful knowledge by actively listening to and observing others as well as asking them pertinent questions.

Analysis of the Data: In the process of providing medical treatment, professionals examine the data that has been gathered to look for trends, outliers, and potential problems. Thinking critically, having clinical experience, and being able to synthesize information are all prerequisites for this step.

Generation of Hypotheses: Healthcare providers generate hypotheses or differential diagnoses based on the results of the study, taking into consideration the most likely conditions that would explain the patient's symptoms. The working theories are comprised of these hypotheses.

Collecting Data and Conducting Tests: In order to validate or invalidate the hypotheses, additional data may be required. The diagnosis may need to be refined after further investigation using studies, testing, or meetings with specialists.

When the facts clearly support a particular condition or group of circumstances, a diagnosis can be made once all of the conditions have been considered. When communicating the diagnosis to the patient and the healthcare team, it is critical to utilize language that is both clear and succinct.

Planning for Treatment Once a diagnosis has been arrived at, the next step in the process is to devise a treatment strategy. This includes making decisions on the most appropriate interventions, drugs, and therapies to treat the diagnosed disease.

Education of the Patient It is important for patients to be informed on their disease, treatment plan, and self-management measures. It is essential to communicate clearly in order to guarantee that the patient understands and complies with instructions.

Monitoring and Following Up: The healthcare practitioners continue to follow up with the patient and monitor their progress, making any necessary adjustments to their treatment plan. Appointments for follow-up care are organized so that the patient's progress can be monitored as they respond to treatment.

In the context of the diagnostic process, clinical reasoning

Clinical reasoning, which refers to the mental process that is used by medical professionals in the course of making clinical choices, includes diagnostic reasoning as one of its subtypes. The integration of clinical knowledge, as well as critical thinking and the ability to solve problems, are essential components of clinical reasoning. Reasoning that is accurate in the clinical setting is necessary for accurate reasoning in diagnostics. The following are important components of clinical reasoning:

Interpretation of the Data Providers are responsible for providing correct interpretations of the data acquired throughout the evaluation. This includes being able to differentiate between normal and aberrant findings, patterns, and trends.

Recognizing Patterns: As they gain more experience, medical professionals improve their capacity to spot patterns in patient data that correspond to a variety of illnesses. This enables diagnosis to be made more quickly and accurately.

Clinical Knowledge It is absolutely necessary to have a strong foundation of clinical knowledge. The biology of diseases, their clinical presentations, and the evidence-based guidelines for diagnosis and treatment are all things that providers need to be familiar with.

Critical Thinking: The ability to analyze, evaluate, and find solutions to problems are examples of critical thinking skills that are essential for clinical reasoning. The providers are responsible for determining the significance of the findings, taking into consideration alternative interpretations, and making decisions based on this information.

Evaluating the Evidence When it comes to making diagnostic and treatment decisions, healthcare providers should base their recommendations on the best available evidence, which includes research, clinical guidelines, and expert consensus.

Clinical reasoning frequently requires the participation of other members of the healthcare team in collaborative endeavors. When making decisions, it might be helpful to get input from professionals including specialists, nurses, and others in the medical field.

Methods for Improving the Quality of Diagnostic Reasoning

The process of enhancing one's abilities in diagnostic thinking is continual. As an AG-ACNP, here are some practices that will help you improve your ability to make correct diagnoses:

Education That Never Stops: Maintain an up-to-date knowledge of the most recent developments in healthcare, including new methods of diagnosis, treatments, and guidelines. To further your education, consider participating in educational gatherings such as conferences, workshops, and even online classes.

Case-based learning involves dissecting difficult patient cases in order to hone diagnostic reasoning skills. This can be done on an individual basis or with other people, opening the door to conversation and a variety of points of view.

Guidelines for Clinical Practice: Familiarize yourself with the guidelines for clinical practice, which include recommendations for diagnosis and treatment that are based on evidence. These recommendations can act as useful references for you to consider when you make decisions.

Mentoring: Seek for mentorship from more experienced healthcare providers, particularly those who are knowledgeable in your area of interest. Your capacity for diagnostic thinking can be considerably improved by gaining knowledge from other people's experiences and perspectives.

Participate in clinical simulations that are modeled after actual contacts with patients when undergoing simulation training. These simulations offer a risk-free setting in which to hone diagnostic reasoning skills through practice and exploration.

Reflective Practice: On a consistent basis, think back on the clinical experiences you've had. Consider some of the situations in which your diagnostic reasoning was questioned or in which you came across some unusual conditions. Examine what aspects performed well and what aspects could want some tweaking.

input & Peer Review: Solicit input from coworkers and other people in your field. Review from peers and feedback that is constructive might be helpful in determining where your diagnostic thinking could use some work.

Interdisciplinary Collaboration: Work closely with other healthcare professionals, like as specialists, nurses, and pharmacists, in order to get a variety of viewpoints and insights into the care of individual patients.

Structured Clinical Reasoning Tools In order to direct and organize your thought process, you should make use of structured clinical reasoning tools and models. Tools such as the "Clinical Reasoning Cycle" might assist you in organizing your thinking in a more logical manner.

Take care of yourself by making sure your body and mind are in good shape through the practice of self-care. Your ability to think clearly might be negatively impacted by factors such as fatigue and stress. Make taking care of yourself a top priority if you want to keep your cognitive abilities at their best.

Obstacles Faced When Using Diagnostic Reasoning

Diagnostic reasoning is a difficult process that involves overcoming a number of obstacles. For the sake of improving diagnostic accuracy, it is vital to be aware of these challenges:

Cognitive Biases Diagnostic errors can be caused by cognitive biases such as confirmation bias (the practice of seeking evidence that confirms prior views) and anchoring bias (the practice of fixating on initial perceptions). Healthcare professionals have an obligation to make concerted efforts to identify and address biases in their practices.

Information That Is Missing There are occasions when medical professionals may not have access to all of the information that is required to provide an accurate diagnosis. In situations like this, they are required to make conclusions based on the information that is currently accessible to them while also taking into consideration whether or not additional evaluation is required.

Disorders that are Extremely Uncommon or Rare Diagnosing disorders that are extremely rare or atypical can be quite difficult. It's possible that healthcare providers don't see certain disorders very often, which makes recognition and diagnosis more challenging.

Acute care settings typically require medical professionals to work under time pressure because of the nature of the service they deliver. This can result in hasty decision-making, which can put a possible damper on the precision of the diagnostic process. It is essential to manage one's time well.

Communication: It is crucial to have effective communication not just within the healthcare team but also with patients. The failure to communicate properly can result in mistakes in diagnosis and treatment.

Patient variables: Patient variables can make the diagnostic procedure more difficult, especially if the patient does not comply with therapy or withholds information. The only way for providers to overcome these obstacles is through clear communication and active participation from patients.

Critical Thinking in the Field of Gerontology

When it comes to diagnosing problems in elderly individuals, various distinct elements come into play, including the following:

Atypical Presentation: A great number of illnesses that affect elderly persons manifest in an unusual way or with only faint symptoms. The professionals who give medical care need to have a high suspicion level and take into account the changes that come with getting older.

Comorbidity: Because elderly people frequently have many chronic diseases, it can be difficult to tell new symptoms apart from those that have already been present in the patient.

Polypharmacy is the practice of taking numerous medications, which can make it difficult to manage a patient's medication regimen and raises the possibility of adverse drug reactions and effects.

Frailty is a disorder that is rather widespread in the aged population and might have an impact on the diagnostic process. Providers are obligated to screen for frailty and take into account how it will affect diagnosis and treatment.

Planning for Future Care: Patients of advanced age may have particular wishes or advance care plans that should be taken into consideration when making diagnostic and therapeutic choices. These preferences need to be taken into consideration by providers.

Functional Status: The functional status of a geriatric patient is an important factor that must be considered during the diagnostic procedure. To identify the effect that a health condition has on activities of daily living, providers need to conduct ADL and IADL assessments.

Geriatric syndromes are conditions that are frequent in the elderly and require specialist diagnosis and therapy procedures. Some examples of these syndromes are dementia, falls, and incontinence.

The Importance of Technology in the Diagnostic Thinking Process

The use of technology is becoming an increasingly crucial factor in diagnostic thinking. Electronic health records, often known as EHRs, allow for easier access to patient information, the results of diagnostic tests, and evidence-based guidelines, all of which contribute to more informed decision-making. In addition, diagnostic technologies including imaging modalities, laboratory analyzers, and molecular testing are continuously advancing, which contributes to an increase in both the accuracy and the speed of diagnosis. AG-ACNPs have a greater reach because to telemedicine and telehealth platforms, which enable them to provide care and diagnostics remotely. This is especially beneficial in locations that are either underserved or rural.

However, the use of technology also offers obstacles, such as the possibility of information overload, incorrect interpretation of data, and worries over cybersecurity. These challenges may arise from the usage of technology. Providers of healthcare must be adept in the use of technology while also having the capacity to think critically and analyze data appropriately.

Acute and Chronic Conditions is the Topic of Chapter 5.

It is absolutely necessary for adult-geriatric acute care nurse practitioners (AG-ACNPs) to have an in-depth knowledge of both acute and chronic medical disorders in order to successfully practice their profession. This chapter will delve into the complexities of these disorders, studying their characteristics as well as the diagnosis and treatment options available for each. Your ability as an AG-ACNP to treat both acute and chronic illnesses in adult and geriatric patients in acute care settings is essential to your ability to provide care that is both holistic and efficient.

Distinction Between Immediately Life-Threatening and Ongoing Conditions

It is essential to gain an understanding of the underlying distinctions that exist between acute and chronic disorders before delving into the specifics of a variety of acute and chronic conditions:

Conditions Classified as Acute Acute conditions are distinguished by the sudden onset of symptoms and the brief length over which they persist. They frequently demand quick attention from a medical professional. Infections, traumatic injuries, or the rapid deterioration of a preexisting chronic condition can all lead to acute illness. Pneumonia, acute myocardial infarction (often known as a heart attack), and appendicitis are all instances of common medical conditions.

Chronic Conditions On the other hand, chronic conditions are defined by a delayed onset of symptoms and often remain for a lengthy period of time, often throughout the lifetime of a person. When treating chronic illnesses, the primary goals of management are symptom management, the prevention of exacerbations, and the improvement of the patient's quality of life. Diabetes, high blood pressure, and chronic obstructive pulmonary disease (often known as COPD) are all examples of common chronic illnesses.

Because of the major differences in how each category approaches assessment, diagnosis, and management, AG-ACNPs need to be highly skilled in differentiating between the two categories.

The Most Frequent Serious Illnesses

1. Acute Respiratory Distress Syndrome (often referred to as ARDS)

The acute respiratory distress syndrome (ARDS) is a severe lung illness that develops as a consequence of an inflammatory reaction in the lungs. This response causes fluid accumulation and interferes with oxygen exchange.

Patients often show with acute dyspnea, fast breathing, and low oxygen levels when they are diagnosed with this condition. In severe situations, the use of mechanical ventilation may be necessary.

The clinical presentation, radiographic abnormalities (for example, bilateral infiltrates on chest X-ray), and low oxygen levels are all taken into consideration when making a diagnosis of ARDS.

The treatment for this condition consists of identifying and treating the underlying cause, providing supportive care such as mechanical ventilation, and managing consequences such as sepsis.

2. Septicemia

Sepsis is a systemic inflammatory response to an infection that can lead to malfunction and failure of organs in the body.

Symptoms include altered mental status, fever, high heart rate, and fast breathing. Other symptoms include an accelerated heart rate. It is possible for this condition to evolve to severe sepsis, which is characterized by organ malfunction, or septic shock, which is characterized by an abnormally low blood pressure.

Clinical indicators, such as symptoms of infection and dysfunction in organ systems, are taken into account while making a diagnosis. In addition to it, laboratory procedures including blood cultures and inflammatory marker levels are utilized.

In terms of management, early detection and intervention are quite important. Antibiotics, fluid resuscitation, vasopressors for hypotension, and supportive care are all part of the treatment for this condition.

3. Acute Coronary Syndrome, Also Known as ACS

ACS refers to a range of cardiac diseases, including unstable angina, non-ST-segment elevation myocardial infarction (also known as NSTEMI), and ST-segment elevation myocardial infarction (also known as STEMI).

Symptoms can range from mild discomfort in the chest (angina) to severe discomfort in the chest, accompanied by shortness of breath and sweating (STEMI).

Clinical examination, abnormalities on an electrocardiogram (ECG), and measuring levels of cardiac biomarkers are all part of the diagnostic process.

Treatment: Treatment for ST-elevation myocardial infarction (STEMI) might vary depending on the individual diagnosis, however it may include antiplatelet medicines, anticoagulants, and reperfusion methods such as percutaneous coronary intervention (PCI).

4. Acute Kidney Injury (often referred to as AKI).

Acute kidney injury (AKI) is a sudden loss of kidney function that can come from a number of different causes, including dehydration, the toxicity of some medications, and infections.

Symptoms may include decreased urine production, fluid retention, electrolyte imbalances, and weariness. Symptoms may also include a decreased urine output.

Alterations in serum creatinine levels and the amount of urine produced are used to form a diagnosis. It is necessary to determine the underlying causes.

Treatment: Treatment consists of investigating and treating the underlying cause of the condition, treating any complications that arise, and in certain cases, administering renal replacement therapy.

5. Embolism of the Pulmonary Artery, Acute (PE)

PE is caused when a blood clot travels to the lungs and causes a blockage in the pulmonary arteries. This results in the symptoms of PE.

The symptoms can vary, but they can include acute chest pain, shortness of breath, and even hemoptysis at times.

Imaging tests such as computed tomography pulmonary angiography (CTPA) and ventilation-perfusion (V/Q) scans are examples of diagnostic techniques that are used in the diagnosis process.

In the management of this condition, treatment consists of anticoagulation to stop the advancement of the clot and supportive care. When the condition is severe, thrombolytic therapy or surgical intervention may be required to treat the patient.

Frequent Ailments of a Chronic Nature

1. Mellitus diabetes insipidus

Diabetes is a chronic metabolic condition that is characterized by increased blood glucose levels due to inadequate insulin synthesis or poor insulin use. These elevated blood glucose levels can be caused by either of these two factors.

Polyuria, also known as excessive urination, polydipsia, or excessive thirst, weight loss, and exhaustion are some of the symptoms that may be experienced.

Blood glucose levels taken while the patient is fasting, oral glucose tolerance tests, or HbA1c readings are used to make the diagnosis of diabetes.

Treatment: Treatment consists of making changes to one's lifestyle (such as one's diet and amount of physical activity), taking oral anti-diabetic drugs, undergoing insulin therapy, and monitoring one's blood glucose levels.

2. Hypertension, most often known as high blood pressure

A chronic illness that is marked by consistently increased blood pressure levels is referred to as hypertension.

Symptoms It's not uncommon for people to have no symptoms of hypertension, yet the condition can develop to complications like stroke, heart disease, and renal issues.

Multiple readings of an abnormally high blood pressure are used to make a diagnosis of hypertension.

Modifications to one's way of life (such as dietary shifts and increased physical activity) and antihypertensive medication are both components of the management strategy.

3. COPD, also known as chronic obstructive pulmonary disease

COPD stands for chronic obstructive pulmonary disease, which refers to a group of lung disorders that include chronic bronchitis and emphysema. It can be recognized by the restricted airflow that it produces.

Symptoms: Some of the most common symptoms are wheezing, shortness of breath, a hacking cough, and production of phlegm.

Spirometry and other tests of pulmonary function, in addition to a clinical evaluation, are used during the diagnostic process.

Cessation of smoking, bronchodilators, corticosteroids, and oxygen therapy are all part of the management of this condition.

4. Heart Failure (HF), often known as

Heart failure is a chronic disorder in which the heart is unable to pump blood adequately, which can cause symptoms such as fluid retention and exhaustion.

Dyspnea, edema, weariness, and a decreased exercise tolerance are some of the symptoms that may be experienced.

The clinical evaluation, echocardiography, and laboratory tests that are performed all contribute to the final diagnosis.

Medication (such as diuretics and ACE inhibitors), changes to one's lifestyle, and, in extreme circumstances, either mechanical circulatory support or heart transplantation are all part of the treatment plan for hypertension.

5. Kidney Disease that is Chronic (CKD)

Chronic kidney disease (CKD) is a disorder that lasts for a long period of time and causes the kidneys to gradually lose their function. This is sometimes caused by other conditions, such as diabetes or hypertension.

Symptoms: The early stages of chronic kidney disease are frequently asymptomatic, but advanced stages of the disease can cause symptoms such as fatigue, fluid retention, and increased creatinine levels.

The glomerular filtration rate (GFR) and the presence of protein in the urine are both important factors to consider when making a diagnosis.

The goal of treatment is to halt the course of chronic kidney disease (CKD), bring blood pressure under control, and treat any problems that may arise.

Methodologies for Treating Acute and Chronic Conditions

As an AG-ACNP, you will regularly come into contact with patients who are suffering from a combination of acute and chronic illnesses. Your strategy for treating these patients should be all-encompassing and centered on the patient:

The first step is to conduct a comprehensive assessment, during which you should take into account both acute and chronic diseases. It is extremely important to pay great attention to any shifts in the patient's symptoms, vital signs, and laboratory results.

Prioritization: Care should be prioritized according to the seriousness and acuteness of the conditions. Take care of the pressing conditions that require immediate attention, such as vital signs that are fluctuating erratically or significant discomfort.

The diagnosis and treatment of acute diseases require quick establishment of a diagnosis and the initiation of treatment that is appropriate for the condition. When dealing with chronic diseases, it is important to evaluate the patient's current management plan, as well as their level of adherence and any possibility for worsening symptoms.

Medication Management In this step, you will go through the patient's medication list and make sure that all of their prescriptions, whether they are for acute or chronic ailments, are optimized and do not cause any adverse drug interactions.

Patient Education: It is important to educate the patient about their diseases, the significance of taking medications as prescribed, making necessary changes to their lifestyle, and developing self-management techniques.

Collaborate with the healthcare team, which should include both primary care doctors and specialists, in order to ensure that acute and chronic illnesses receive coordinated care.

Long-Term Planning It is important to participate in long-term planning while dealing with chronic illnesses. The planning should center on the prevention of exacerbations, complications, and readmissions to the hospital.

Follow-Up Appointments at Regular Intervals: It is important to assess the patient's progress at regular intervals, adjust treatment as necessary, and handle any new acute or chronic problems as they arise.

Taking into Account Certain Specifics Regarding Elderly Patients

Patients who are elderly frequently appear with a complicated set of medical demands, which may include many chronic illnesses. When it comes to the management of acute and chronic illnesses in this population, certain special concerns should be taken into account:

Due to the prevalence of many chronic illnesses among elderly people, polypharmacy is a risk factor for these patients. Review their current prescription list, take into consideration the possibility of deprescribing any superfluous drugs, and handle any possible drug interactions.

Cognitive function, functional status, and the influence of the patient's chronic diseases on their day-to-day life should all be evaluated as part of a comprehensive assessment. Adapt management so as to get the highest possible quality of life.

Geriatric Syndromes: It is important to be on the lookout for geriatric syndromes, such as frailty, falls, and incontinence, because they can influence the progression of both acute and chronic illnesses.

dialogues about advance care planning, end-of-life wishes, and care goals should be included in advance care planning dialogues. These conversations are absolutely necessary in order to provide care that is focussed on the patient.

Multidisciplinary Collaboration: When addressing the specific requirements of geriatric patients, it is important to work together with geriatricians, as well as occupational therapists, physical therapists, and social workers.

Putting an Emphasis on Preventive Care: Put an emphasis on preventive care to lower the risk of acute diseases and to minimize the exacerbation of chronic ailments.

Pharmacology and Medication Management are the Topics of Chapter 6.

Adult-Gerontology Acute Care Nurse Practitioners, often known as AG-ACNPs, place a significant emphasis on pharmacology and the administration of medications as part of their clinical duties. This chapter presents a comprehensive analysis of pharmacology, including topics such as drug classifications, the fundamentals of medication management, and unique concerns that should be taken into account while prescribing and providing medication to adult and elderly patients in acute care settings.

Primordial Principles of Pharmacology

Both pharmacokinetics and pharmacodynamics need to be considered.

In order to manage medications in a way that is both safe and effective, it is necessary to have a fundamental understanding of pharmacokinetics and pharmacodynamics.

A drug's absorption, distribution, metabolism, and elimination (ADME) are all components of its pharmacokinetics. Pharmacokinetics is the study of how medications are processed by the body. The bioavailability of the drug, its half-life, and its clearance are all important topics.

Pharmacodynamics refers to the process through which medications produce their desired effects on the body. It takes into account things like drug receptors, dose-response correlations, and mechanisms of action.

Classes of Drugs

The AG-ACNP field is exposed to a diverse array of pharmacological classes, each of which has its own set of characteristics and indications. The following are examples of common drug classes:

Antibiotics are necessary for the treatment of bacterial infections in acute care settings. Common types of antibiotics include penicillins, cephalosporins, and fluoroquinolones.

Cardiovascular Medications: These medications include anti-arrhythmics, anti-coagulants, and anti-hypertensives, and they are used to control problems related to the heart.

Analgesics: Pain management is a critical component of therapy, and analgesics such as opioids, non-steroidal anti-inflammatory medications (NSAIDs), and acetaminophen are used to treat the discomfort that patients experience.

Insulin, metformin, and sulfonylureas are examples of diabetes drugs that are frequently used for the treatment and management of the condition known as diabetes.

Medication for the Respiratory System Bronchodilators and corticosteroids are necessary for the effective management of respiratory disorders such asthma and chronic obstructive pulmonary disease (COPD).

Polypharmacy as well as Reconciliation of Medications

Patients of all ages who are coping with various chronic diseases are more likely to engage in polypharmacy, which refers to the use of many medications at the same time. It is essential to do medication reconciliation, also known as the process of evaluating and keeping the prescription list up to date, in order to reduce the risk of dangerous drug interactions and to enhance patient safety.

Acute Care Settings' Medication Management and Administration

The Administration of Medication

It is the responsibility of AG-ACNPs to administer drugs, including those given intravenously (IV), which calls for specialized knowledge and abilities. Calculating the appropriate dosage, preparing the drug, and educating the patient are three important aspects to take into account before administering medication.

Security of Medication

Errors in medication can have devastating effects for patients. The use of barcode scanning, the "five rights" of medicine administration (the right patient, the right medication, the right dose, the right route, and the right time), and cultivating a culture of safety within healthcare institutions are all strategies that can improve the safety of medication.

A look at pharmacogenetics

The field of pharmacogenetics investigates how the genetic make-up of an individual can influence how they react to certain drugs. One area of personalized medicine that is experiencing rapid expansion is the practice of customizing pharmacological therapy based on a patient's genetic profile.

As an AG-ACNP, you are able to prescribe medication.

AG-ACNPs have the ability to prescribe a wide variety of drugs because they have the prescriptive power to do so. The following are important principles for safe and successful prescribing:

Evidence-based practice states that prescribing decisions should be based on the most compelling evidence currently available, in addition to clinical standards and the specific requirements of the individual patient.

Care that is centered on the patient involves engaging in collaborative decision-making with the patient, taking into account the patient's preferences, goals, and concerns.

In the management of polypharmacy, it is important to be aware of the possibility of adverse drug interactions, the accumulation of side effects, and the overall burden of medicine for patients who suffer from many chronic illnesses.

Patient Education Regarding Medication It is important to educate patients on their medications in depth, including how to take them, any potential adverse effects, and how important it is to take them as prescribed.

When prescribing opioids for pain management, it is important to follow best practices in order to reduce the risk of opioid misuse, abuse, and overdose.

Compliance with Regulations It is imperative that compliance with state and federal regulations that govern controlled substances and prescription drug monitoring programs is maintained.

Important Considerations for the Medication of Elderly Patients

Geriatric people may require special considerations with regard to medication, including the following:

Changes in Pharmacokinetics: Changes in metabolism and clearance that are associated with aging can have an impact on medication dosing and pharmacokinetics. Drugs that are removed by the kidneys could require certain adjustments.

Geriatric people are more prone to take many drugs, which increases the risk of side effects and drug interactions. This practice is referred to as polypharmacy. Reviews of medications are very important.

Consider the patient's state of frailty, since this can play a role in the drug that is prescribed and the dosage that is given.

Cognitive Function: When prescribing, it is important to evaluate a patient's cognitive function because patients who have cognitive impairments may have trouble following complicated prescription schedules.

Beers Criteria: Familiarize yourself with the Beers Criteria, which provide advise on drugs that should be avoided or taken with caution in older persons.

They may be found here. Beers Criteria: Familiarize yourself with the Beers Criteria.

The Importance of Correctly Taking Medications

It is absolutely necessary to do a process known as medication reconciliation, which entails producing a list of all the medications that a patient is currently taking that is as exact as it can possibly be, in order to minimize the risk of medication errors and maximize the safety of the patient. The following are important aspects of the medication reconciliation process:

Reviewing the patient's current medication list, which may include prescription drugs, over-the-counter drugs, herbal supplements, and vitamin and mineral supplements, is part of the process of obtaining a complete medication history for the patient.

Comparing Medication Lists The AG-ACNP needs to check the patient's current medication list with the one that was prescribed, looking for any differences or omissions between the two.

Review of Medication Assess whether or not each medication is appropriate for the patient by taking into account their diagnosis, their present state of health, and any possible drug interactions.

Education Regarding Medication It is important to provide the patient with a thorough education regarding their drugs. This education should cover dosing instructions, potential adverse effects, and the significance of adhering to their medication regimen.

The Administration of Medications During Hospice and Palliative Care

In end-of-life care, when drug management takes on a particularly significant role, AG-ACNPs frequently play an important and sometimes pivotal role. The management of symptoms, the improvement of quality of life, and the maintenance of the patient's comfort are all goals. The following are important things to keep in mind regarding medication administration during end-of-life care:

Medications for Palliative Care: Medications to treat pain and symptoms, like opioids and sedatives, are frequently used to enhance a patient's comfort as part of palliative care.

Engage in conversations regarding advance care planning, which should include the usage of particular medications or interventions, as well as the patient's goals and preferences.

Education of the Family and Caregivers It is important to educate the family members and caregivers on the medications that are being used, what their purpose is, and any possible adverse effects that they may have.

Emotional Support: It is important to acknowledge the emotional and psychological aspects of end-of-life care and to offer support to both patients and the families of those patients.

Ethical Considerations: It is important to be aware of the ethical issues that are associated to the management of medication in end-of-life care. These ethical issues include the principles of autonomy, beneficence, and non-maleficence.

Management of Acute and Critical Care Patients is the topic of Chapter 7.

The Adult-Gerontology Acute Care Nurse Practitioner (AG-ACNP) job has a primary emphasis on the management of patients receiving acute and critical care services. This chapter presents a comprehensive overview of the skills, knowledge, and methods required to provide high-quality treatment to patients in acute and critical care settings. Particular attention is paid to the specific requirements of geriatric populations as well as adult populations of all ages.

An Introduction to the Management of Acute and Critical Care

Patients with life-threatening diseases, serious injuries, or complex medical difficulties are evaluated, treated, and given continued care as part of the treatment of acute and critical care. In these types of healthcare facilities, AG-ACNPs are essential members of the caregiving staff, playing an essential part in maximizing positive patient outcomes and assuring the provision of care that is both evidence-based and patient-centered.

Management of Acute and Critical Care Based on Core Principles

1. Immediate Evaluation and Prioritization of Needs

It is absolutely necessary to be able to conduct a patient assessment that is both quick and thorough. This involves analyzing the patient's airway, breathing, circulation, and disability (also known as the ABCDs), as well as locating conditions that are potentially fatal.

It is imperative that care be prioritized in accordance with the condition of the patient as well as the gravity of their disease or injury. The Glasgow Coma Scale and the Sequential Organ Failure Assessment (SOFA) score are two examples of useful instruments that can be utilized to assist in the prioritization process.

2. Management of the Airway

Maintaining a clear airway should be your number one concern. AG-ACNPs are required to have expertise in a variety of procedures, such as intubation and the utilization of advanced airway devices, in order to establish and maintain airway patency.

When treating elderly patients, it is important to keep in mind the potential difficulties that may arise from age-related changes in the structure of the airways as well as cognitive decline.

3. Monitoring of the Hemodynamic State

It is extremely important to monitor and take care of a patient's hemodynamic state. Checking the patient's blood pressure, heart rate, cardiac output, and central venous pressure are all part of this process.

When treating elderly patients, it is important to keep an eye out for orthostatic variations in blood pressure and heart rate, as well as the effect that drugs have on the patient's hemodynamics.

4. Procedures That Are Invasive

Invasive operations such as the insertion of a chest tube, a central line, or an arterial line can be carried out by AG-ACNPs, or they can help in their performance.

Technique and monitoring that are executed with extreme caution are necessities while dealing with elderly individuals because of the increased risk of skin fragility and infection.

5. The Pharmacological Administration

A crucial competence is the ability to administer medication competently, both orally and intravenously, including other medications. A knowledge of vasoactive medicines, sedatives, analgesics, and antimicrobials is included in this.

Be aware of the specific pharmacokinetic and pharmacodynamic changes that occur in elderly patients, since these changes can have an effect on the dosage and reaction to medications.

6. Collaboration across multiple disciplines

In intensive care settings, collaboration with a multidisciplinary healthcare team, consisting of intensivists, surgeons, nurses, respiratory therapists, and pharmacists, is absolutely necessary in order to provide the highest possible level of care to patients.

In the management of elderly patients who have several complex conditions, it is important to acknowledge the necessity of interprofessional care coordination.

The Management of Severe and Life-Threatening Conditions

1. Septic shock and septic septicemia

Sepsis is a disorder that poses a significant risk to the patient's life and requires rapid diagnosis and treatment. The screening, evaluation, and management of sepsis should be well within the AG-ACNPs' capabilities.

When dealing with elderly patients, one must take into account the difficulties of diagnosing sepsis in the presence of various comorbidities as well as the age-related changes in vital signs.

2. Acute Respiratory Distress Syndrome (often referred to as ARDS)

The acute respiratory distress syndrome (ARDS) is a life-threatening disorder marked by severe hypoxemia. The early detection of the condition and the provision of supportive care, which may include the use of mechanical ventilation, are essential components of management.

Examine elderly individuals for the possible presence of co-existing diseases as well as abnormalities in lung function that are associated with advancing age.

3. Treatment of Trauma and Accidental Injuries

It is possible for AG-ACNPs to take part in the treatment of patients who have suffered traumatic injuries, such as those brought on by accidents or falls. Important skills include assessment of trauma, cardiopulmonary resuscitation, and surgical intervention.

When caring for elderly patients, it is important to take into consideration the risk of injury that is related with falling and fragility fractures. It is necessary to exercise extreme caution.

4. Emergencies Related to the Heart

In order to effectively manage cardiac crises, such as acute myocardial infarction (also known as AMI) and cardiac arrhythmias, prompt assessment and intervention are required. In some cases, medical interventions like percutaneous coronary intervention (PCI) may be required.

Patients who are elderly have an increased likelihood of experiencing a cardiac episode. Changes in the cardiovascular system that are associated with aging should be taken into consideration during assessment.

5. Emergencies Related to the Nervous System

Patients who are experiencing neurological emergencies such as a stroke or traumatic brain damage may be treated by AG-ACNPs. The importance of rapid assessment, imaging, and intervention cannot be overstated.

When caring for elderly patients, it is important to keep in mind the danger of falls that could result in traumatic brain injuries as well as the possibility of delayed presentation of stroke symptoms.

6. Emergencies Related to the Digestive System and the Abdomen

A fast diagnosis and treatment are required for conditions such as bleeding in the gastrointestinal tract, acute pancreatitis, and bowel blockage. The

AG-ACNPs ought to be competent in the evaluation and management of abdominal discomfort as well as emergency situations.

Recognize the possibility for atypical presentations of abdominal illnesses in elderly patients, as well as the influence of age-related changes on gastrointestinal function.

Critical Care for the Elderly: Additional Important Considerations

Patients in critical care who are elderly frequently have more complicated comorbidities and specific need for care. The following are examples of special considerations:

Assessing frailty requires that you be aware of the condition, which can have an effect on a patient's capacity to endure critical care interventions. Use tools such as the Clinical Frailty Scale to conduct an assessment of frailty.

Advance Care Planning: Have conversations with patients about advance care planning, and make it a priority to ensure that the patient's values and desires are taken into account in all decisions regarding critical care.

Cognitive Impairment It is important to remain vigilant for cognitive impairment, which can have an effect on a patient's capacity to engage in their own care and to make decisions.

Polypharmacy refers to the practice of elderly persons taking numerous drugs, which might increase the likelihood of harmful drug interactions and side effects. Reviews of medications are very important.

Mobility and Rehabilitation It is important to promote early mobility and rehabilitation in geriatric patients who are receiving critical care in order to forestall a decline in their functional status.

Concerns Regarding Ethical Behavior in Intensive Care

The context of critical care frequently gives rise to difficult ethical questions. The ethical concepts of justice, beneficence, non-maleficence, and autonomy are some of the topics that an AG-ACNP should be conversant with.

Consider making decisions on end-of-life care, such as having conversations about do-not-resuscitate (DNR) orders, discontinuing artificial life support, and receiving palliative care.

Enhancement of Quality and Protection of Patients

In settings dealing with critical care, encourage a culture that focuses on the continual improvement of patient safety and quality. Take part in efforts that aim to reduce the number of infections that are related with healthcare, as well as drug errors and other bad events.

Participate in activities such as incident reporting and root cause analysis in order to locate care delivery areas that could use some tweaking.

The Structures of Healthcare Organizations and Their Policies

The Adult-Gerontology Acute Care Nurse Practitioners (AG-ACNPs) have a considerable impact on the healthcare landscape, particularly with regard to the policies and systems that are a part of it. This chapter examines the organization of healthcare systems, healthcare policy, and the role of AG-ACNPs in navigating and influencing these systems so that adult and geriatric patients in acute care settings can receive high-quality care.

A Brief Introduction to Healthcare Organizations and Policy

The term "healthcare system" refers to a complex network of institutions, providers, payers, and rules that are meant to provide medical care to an entire population. In the context of healthcare, "healthcare policy" refers to the collection of laws, regulations, and guidelines that direct the administration of healthcare systems. AG-ACNPs function within this complex environment, and in order to deliver good treatment, they need to have a solid understanding of its dynamics.

The Healthcare System in the United States

The Organization of the Health Care System in the United States

The public and private sectors work together in tandem to form the foundation of the healthcare system in the United States. It is made up of a few essential parts, namely:

Both public and private insurance options are available to patients. Patients may obtain coverage through public programs such as Medicare and

Medicaid, or they may enroll in a private insurance plan through their work or independently.

Hospitals and other healthcare facilities A network of hospitals, outpatient clinics, long-term care institutions, and other types of venues are responsible for providing medical care to patients.

Providers of Healthcare include general practitioners, nurse practitioners, registered nurses, specialists, allied health workers, and other medical professionals.

Manufacturers create medications, medical devices, and treatments that are employed in the healthcare industry. Pharmaceutical and medical device companies fall under this category.

Oversight by the Government A number of federal and state agencies, such as the Centers for Medicare & Medicaid Services (CMS) and the Food and Drug Administration (FDA), are responsible for the regulation and oversight of the healthcare industry.

Access to Medical Care

Having access to various medical treatments is a major area of concern. The capacity of an individual to gain access to medical care is influenced by a variety of factors, including their geographical location, socioeconomic standing, and insurance coverage. AG-ACNPs frequently face differences in access, which may have an impact on the results of their patients.

Models for the Provision of Healthcare

The provision of medical care can be accomplished through a variety of different methods, including fee-for-service and value-based care, for example. Because these models can have an effect on both the reimbursement and the delivery of patient care, it is essential for an AG-ACNP to have a solid understanding of them.

Policy and Regulation in the Healthcare Industry

The Medicare and Medicaid programs

Both Medicare and Medicaid are insurance programs that are funded by the government and play an important position in the healthcare system, particularly for people who are older:

Medicare is a federal program that offers medical coverage to those who are 65 years old or older, as well as younger people who have certain disabilities. AG-ACNPs frequently provide care for patients who are enrolled in Medicare.

Medicaid is a program that is run jointly by the federal government and the states, and it provides medical coverage to individuals and families with low incomes. Medicaid is the primary source of funding for the medical care of a significant number of elderly patients.

Reforms in Health Care

The Affordable Care Act (ACA) is one example of an effort to change the healthcare system with the goals of increasing access to healthcare, improving the quality of care provided, and bringing down prices. AG-ACNPs are required to maintain a level of knowledge on ever-changing healthcare policies and the effect those policies have on patient care.

Measures of Quality and Reporting on Their Status

The level of reimbursement in value-based care models is directly related to quality and performance measures. The reporting of data on these measures is mandatory for healthcare organizations and providers. In order to fulfill these standards, AG-ACNPs are frequently participating in efforts aimed at quality improvement.

The Breadth of Our Work

The range of our activities The scope of services that AG-ACNPs are permitted to deliver is governed by rules. These rules can limit the liberty of nurse practitioners in the way they provide care, and they differ from state to state.

AG-ACNPs and Their Importance in the Healthcare System and Policy

The following are some of the ways in which AG-ACNPs play an important role in healthcare systems and policy:

1. Providing Treatment and Care to Individual Patients

AG-ACNPs are typically found working in the most direct patient care settings. Within the context of acute care settings, they are responsible for the diagnosis, treatment, and management of complex acute and chronic illnesses in adult and geriatric patients.

2. Working in Partnership with Multidisciplinary Teams

When it comes to providing comprehensive and coordinated treatment in acute care settings, AG-ACNPs collaborate closely with physicians, nurses, specialists, pharmacists, and other medical professionals to meet patient needs.

3. Serving as an Advocate for Patients

The role of the AG-ACNP is to act as an advocate for their patients, making certain that their patients receive the necessary care and that their beliefs and preferences are respected.

4. Utilizing Practices That Are Backed By Evidence

When making clinical judgments, AG-ACNPs rely on evidence-based recommendations; as a result, the care they provide is grounded in the most recent research and industry standards.

5. Understanding and Complying with the Necessary Regulations

AG-ACNPs are required to traverse a complicated regulatory landscape in the healthcare industry, which includes payment criteria, state legislation governing the scope of practice, and quality reporting requirements.

6. Participating in Efforts to Improve Quality

One of the most important responsibilities is to take part in various efforts aimed at quality improvement. AG-ACNPs provide significant contributions to the enhancement of care quality, patient safety, and the outcomes of healthcare.

7. Advancing the Cause of Preventive Care

It is absolutely necessary to encourage preventative treatment in order to lessen the impact of chronic diseases and to keep patients healthy. AG-ACNPs highlight the significance of preventative measures such as vaccines, screenings, and changes in lifestyle.

Both difficulties and prospects are involved.

In terms of healthcare systems and policy, AG-ACNPs confront a variety of difficulties and opportunities, including the following:

1. Obstacles Created by Regulations

The legislation governing the scope of practice can differ greatly from one state to another, which prevents AG-ACNPs from making full use of their talents and knowledge. Ongoing advocacy work is being done in order to overcome these obstacles.

2. Changing Methods of Financial Compensation

Alterations to reimbursement models, such as value-based care, create possibilities and problems for geriatric acute care nurse practitioners (AG-ACNPs). These models need placing an emphasis on quality, efficacy, and the final results for the patient.

3. Developments and Advances in Technology

There are numerous ways in which the incorporation of technology into healthcare, such as electronic health records (EHRs) and telemedicine, can improve the delivery of care and the level of patient participation.

4. Addressing Inequalities in Health Care Provision

AG-ACNPs are obligated to address healthcare inequities, particularly those that exist in minority and underserved populations. Care and outreach initiatives that are culturally appropriate are absolutely necessary.

5. Having an Impact on Health Care Policy

Advocates, AG-ACNPs can participate in professional groups and participate in conversations about healthcare reform to increase their chances of having an impact on healthcare policy.

Professional Development for Adult-Gerontology Acute Care Nurse Practitioners (AG-ACNPs) is the topic of discussion in Chapter 9.

Adult-Gerontology Acute Care Nurse Practitioners (AG-ACNPs) are required to continue their education and training throughout their whole careers as nurse practitioners in acute care settings. This chapter examines the significance of continuous professional development, the approaches that can be taken to accomplish it, and the resources that AG-ACNPs can make use of to improve their abilities, knowledge, and career prospects.

An Introduction to Continuing Education and Professional Development

Development of one's professional abilities, knowledge, and competence is the primary goal of professional development, which is a dynamic process that includes a wide variety of activities and tactics. In order for AG-ACNPs to provide high-quality treatment, keep up with the latest evidence-based techniques, and move ahead in their careers, they need to engage in ongoing professional development.

The Importance of Continuing Education for Agricultural and Veterinary Nurse Practitioners

Clinical Competence: AG-ACNPs must engage in continuous education in order to maintain their clinical competence, which is the ability to render correct diagnoses and provide the highest possible level of care to adult and geriatric patients who are hospitalized.

Adaptation to Change: The area of healthcare is always changing, and as a result, new treatments, technology, and standards are constantly being developed. The ability to adjust to these changes is helped for AG-ACNPs via professional development.

Career Progression If you can show that you are dedicated to your professional development, you may be able to advance your career in ways such as taking on leadership roles or specializing in a particular subfield of acute care.

Patient Safety: To ensure patient safety, it is critical to remain current with both established best practices and cutting-edge research. Those AG-ACNPs who participate in continuing education activities lead to a reduction in medical mistakes and an improvement in patient outcomes.

Interprofessional Collaboration The healthcare industry is known for its emphasis on teamwork, and continuing one's education is one way to improve one's ability to communicate effectively and work effectively with other healthcare professionals.

Leadership and Advocacy: Professional development provides AG-ACNPs with the knowledge and skills essential to advocate for patients, influence policy, and undertake leadership roles within healthcare organizations. This equips them to take on leadership responsibilities.

Techniques for Furthering One's Professional Career

In order to further their professional growth, AG-ACNPs may choose from a variety of approaches, including the following:

1. Education That Never Stops

One of the most important ways to stay current on clinical practices, recommendations, and emerging research is to participate in continuing education opportunities such as classes, workshops, and conferences.

Courses specializing in acute care and gerontology that are geared specifically toward AG-ACNPs are offered by a wide variety of professional organizations and educational institutions.

2. The Most Recent Accreditations

The pursuit of advanced certifications, such as the AG-ACNP certification, displays a commitment to increasing one's level of competence and furthering one's career.

Career chances can be increased by obtaining specialized qualifications in fields such as critical care, cardiology, or palliative care, among others.

3. Preceptorship and Mentorship for New Employees

The formation of mentor-mentee relationships with experienced AG-ACNPs can provide assistance and insights that are of incalculable value.

By acting as preceptors for inexperienced AG-ACNPs or nursing students, experienced practitioners are able to pass on their knowledge and skills to the next generation of healthcare professionals.

4. Academic Investigations and Publications

One's comprehension of evidence-based practice can be improved by participating in research initiatives and publishing their findings in publications that are reviewed by their peers.

Participation in research or quality improvement programs can also contribute to improvements in patient care, so it's important to look for those opportunities.

5. Making connections

Opportunities for networking and working together can be found by becoming a member of professional organizations such as the American Association of Critical-Care Nurses (AACN) or the Gerontological Advanced Practice Nurses Association (GAPNA).

Building professional relationships can result in the acquisition of new employment prospects, partnerships on research initiatives, and access to a variety of resources.

6. Introspection and Evaluation of Oneself

A crucial tool for one's professional development is periodic self-evaluation, which should include contemplation on both one's existing skills and opportunities for growth.

When building a tailored development plan, it is helpful to first identify areas in which growth is needed and then to create precise goals for that progress.

Instruments for One's Own Professional Growth

On their path toward professional growth, AG-ACNPs can benefit from a variety of tools and resources, including the following:

1. Trade and Professional Associations

Educational tools, chances to network with other professionals, and rules for professional practice can be found on the websites of organizations such as the American Nurses Association (ANA), the AACN, and the GAPNA.

These organizations welcome AG-ACNPs to join and provide them with access to their membership benefits, which include essential content such as clinical practice guidelines and research.

2. Methods of Instruction Conducted Online

Coursera, edX, and Nurse.com are just a few of the many online educational platforms that provide a diverse selection of courses, webinars, and other instructional content to medical professionals.

These platforms offer flexibility, which enables AG-ACNPs to learn at their own pace, making the most of their time.

3. Seminars, Conventions, and Workshops

Attending conferences and workshops centered on acute care and gerontology is an efficient approach to stay up to date with the latest best practices. Examples of such conferences and workshops include the AACN National Teaching Institute & Critical Care Exposition.

These events offer the chance to get knowledge from industry professionals and to network with colleagues.

4. Practice in a Clinical Setting

By utilizing clinical simulation programs, advanced practice nurse practitioners (AG-ACNPs) are able to practice and improve their clinical abilities in a safe setting.

Simulations can be modified to reflect the specific issues and circumstances that are encountered in clinical practice.

5. Guidelines and Protocols for Clinical Practice

It is absolutely necessary for evidence-based practice to maintain a level of familiarity with the most recent clinical recommendations and procedures, such as those issued by the Society of Critical Care Medicine (SCCM) and the American College of Cardiology (ACC).

The AG-ACNPs ought to consult these resources on a consistent basis in order to direct their clinical judgments.

6. Newspapers, magazines, and other publications

The availability of academic journals, such as the American Journal of Critical Care (AJCC) and the Journal of Gerontological Nursing, makes it possible to gain access to a plethora of research and information that may be used to inform practice.

Reading research publications and being able to provide an informed critique of them is a vital ability for AG-ACNPs.

Taking Into Account Ethical and Legal Implications

Ethical and legal standards are used as a compass to direct professional progress.

1. Capacity for Ongoing Improvement

The ethical duty of AG-ACNPs to maintain their competence in their practice comes with the territory. Continuous education and critical reflection on one's own performance are required here.

When it comes time to renew a nursing license or keep a certification current, state nursing boards and certifying bodies frequently demand a certain minimum number of continuing education hours.

2. Privacy of the Patient

The standards outlined in the Health Insurance Portability and Accountability Act (HIPAA) must be followed by AG-ACNPs at all times, especially when using online learning platforms, taking part in online communities or forums, and communicating with other users online.

When discussing individual patients' cases, it is important to not disclose any identifiable patient information.

3. Methods of Conducting Ethical Research

If they are involved in research, AG-ACNPs are required to abide by the ethical principles that govern the conduct of research. These principles require them to get participants' informed consent and preserve both their rights and their well-being.

When it comes to publicizing the results of research, ethical issues take precedence.

Continuing One's Education and Training During the Course of a Career

Continuing one's education and training throughout one's career as an AG-ACNP is an essential component of professional development.

Early Stages of Professional Development

During the beginning of their careers, a focus is placed on the acquisition of basic skills, the development of clinical expertise, and the construction of a solid knowledge base by AG-ACNPs.

At this point in time, guidance from an experienced individual is quite beneficial.

Growth and Change in One's Mid-Career

AG-ACNPs who have reached the middle of their careers frequently look for opportunities to specialize or take on leadership roles.

Steps often consist of pursuing more advanced qualifications and actively participating in quality improvement projects.

Late-Career Advancement of One's Career

Later on in their careers, AG-ACNPs may decide to move into areas related to teaching, research, or administrative work.

The transmission of information to the subsequent generation of practitioners should be a top focus.

Getting Ready for a Prosperous Career as an Adult-Gerontology Acute Care Nurse Practitioner (AG-ACNP) is the Topic of Chapter 10.

Getting ready for a successful career as an Adult-Gerontology Acute Care Nurse Practitioner (AG-ACNP) is a multi-step process that requires careful planning, a dedication to professional development, and continual education. This chapter examines the fundamental processes and strategies that will help AG-ACNPs flourish in their profession, give high-quality care to adult and elderly patients in acute care settings, and manage the intricacies of the healthcare industry. These stages and strategies will help AG-ACNPs deliver high-quality care to adult and geriatric patients in acute care settings.

A Step-by-Step Guide to Getting Ready for Success

To be successful in the role of an AG-ACNP, you will need to make an active and ongoing effort to improve your clinical competence, uphold ethical standards, and participate in professional development. AG-ACNPs have the ability to improve patient care while also fostering a pleasant and fulfilling career if they rigorously prepare for the responsibilities and obstacles associated with the profession.

The Building Blocks of Victory

1. Formal Education and Professional Accreditation

A strong educational foundation is the starting point for any journey toward becoming a successful AG-ACNP. They graduate with a Master of Science in Nursing (MSN) or a Doctor of Nursing Practice (DNP), specializing in adult-gerontology acute care from an accredited institution.

The most important step is to become certified as an AG-ACNP by reputable organizations like the American Association of Critical-Care Nurses (AACN) or the American Nurses Credentialing Center (ANCC). The achievement of certification demonstrates clinical skill and competence.

2. A valid license

In order to practice, advanced practice nurse practitioners (AG-ACNPs) need to get a state license as an advanced practice registered nurse (APRN). The prerequisites for obtaining a license are different in each state, but often include of filling out an application, passing a national certification exam, and fulfilling any required hours of continuing education.

Maintaining one's practice privileges requires keeping one's license in good standing at all times. AG-ACNPs are responsible for keeping their licenses current and renewing them as necessary by respective state boards.

3. Capability in the Clinical Setting

The foundation of success is found in clinical competence. The clinical knowledge, skills, and proficiencies of AG-ACNPs should be kept current through periodic self-assessment, as well as through continuing education, practical experience, and shadowing opportunities.

Gaining clinical skill is significantly facilitated by participating in mentoring and preceptorship programs with more seasoned practitioners.

Techniques for Achieving Victory on the Field

1. Continuous Continuing Education and Training

Learning throughout one's entire life should be a top priority for successful AG-ACNPs, and they should participate in ongoing professional development. This entails participating in events such as conferences, workshops, and classes, as well as earning advanced certifications.

The use of online learning platforms, clinical simulation, and participation in research initiatives are a few other approaches to increase one's level of knowledge.

2. Ethical Standards of Conduct

A non-negotiable requirement for one's success is the upholding of ethical standards. The AG-ACNP is expected to respect ethical standards and place patient safety, confidentiality, and autonomy at the forefront of their practice.

It is absolutely necessary to adhere to professional ethical guidelines while also honoring the rights of patients and receiving their informed permission.

3. Working Together Effectively in Teams

One of the most telling indicators of success is successful collaboration with interprofessional teams. In order to provide complete care, AG-ACNPs need to be able to interact effectively with other healthcare professionals, including physicians, nurses, therapists, and others.

It is essential to maintain a commitment to communication that is both pen and polite.

4. Abilities in Leadership

Those who work in the field of geriatrics and want to enhance their careers should work on developing their leadership skills. Taking the initiative, finding solutions to problems, and advocating for patients are all essential components of leadership.

Opportunities for leadership can be found by joining professional groups and taking part in projects to improve quality.

5. Capacity for Change

Adaptability is essential to achieve success in acute care nursing. The ability to adapt to shifting patient requirements, evolving clinical guidelines, and rapid technological development is a requirement for AG-ACNPs.

Important is a mindset that is open to incorporating new ideas, procedures, and tools.

Developing a Promising Professional Career

1. Domain-Specific Knowledge and Experience

A person in the acute care field who wants to distinguish themselves and develop a successful career should consider specialization. Additional certifications, such as those in cardiology, critical care, or neurology, are open to AG-ACNPs who wish to further their careers.

Becoming a specialist in a certain area might open doors to leadership positions and other opportunities for advancement.

2. Making Connections and Seeking Advice

Building professional relationships is an effective strategy for advancing one's career. AG-ACNPs are strongly encouraged to engage in active participation in professional organizations, attendance at conferences, and networking with colleagues in their area.

The formation of mentor-mentee relationships provides direction and opportunities for insight into professional development.

3. Institutions of Learning and Instruction

A potential route to job growth is making the transition into education and teaching roles, whether in the academic world or in clinical education.

AG-ACNPs have the ability to work in the clinical setting as lecturers, preceptors, or instructors for nursing students.

4. Academic Work and Investigative Work

Participation in research and scholarly activities not only makes a contribution to the development of nursing as a profession but also provides opportunities for professional advancement.

Participating in scholarly activities can be accomplished through activities such as collaborating on research projects, publishing findings, and presenting at conferences.

Managing Difficulties While Attempting to Keep Your Balance

1. Methods to Prevent Burnout

The provision of acute care can be taxing, and acute care nurse practitioners (AG-ACNPs) need to be diligent about preventing burnout. Strategies consist of establishing limits, taking breaks at regular intervals, and engaging in self-care practices.

It can be useful to participate in stress-reduction activities such as mindfulness meditation or physical activity.

2. Obstacles of a Legal and Ethical Nature

In the practice of acute care, there is the potential for legal and ethical complications. AG-ACNPs are expected to maintain current knowledge of healthcare regulations, adhere to professional codes of ethics, and seek qualified legal counsel when appropriate.

In order to effectively address such difficulties, it is essential to uphold a commitment to ethical practice.

3. Finding a Good Balance Between Work and Life

Achieving a healthy balance between one's professional and personal life is critical to one's long-term success. It is important for AG-ACNPs to create a timetable that makes room for both personal development and professional advancement.

Maintaining a healthy work-life balance requires consistent introspection and assessment.

4. Influence on Public Policy and Advocacy

Participating in advocacy and policy work is one strategy for addressing issues that have been identified within the healthcare system. The AG-ACNPs have the ability to have an impact on healthcare policy, to advocate for patient rights, and to advance nursing practice rights.

It is possible to make a difference by becoming a member of professional organizations and taking part in advocacy activities.

The Path to Certification for Adult-Gerontology Acute Care Nurse Practitioners (AG-ACNPs) is the Topic of Chapter 11 of this Book.

In order to advance one's career as an Adult-Gerontology Acute Care Nurse Practitioner (AG-ACNP), certification is an absolutely necessary step. This chapter goes into the process of becoming certified as an AG-ACNP, beginning with the decision to become certified and continuing through the preparation, examination, and continuing certification requirements. Those who aspire to flourish in this specialized nursing profession need to have a solid understanding of this path in order to get there.

An Overview of the AG-ACNP Certification Process

The AG-ACNP certification is a recognized acknowledgement of a nurse practitioner's ability in providing advanced care to adult and geriatric patients in acute care settings. The certification is awarded by the American College of Nurse Practitioners. In this difficult industry, having a certification demonstrates that you are committed to becoming the best you can be and to maintaining the highest possible standards of professional conduct.

Why Should One Attempt to Obtain AG-ACNP Certification?

Certification provides a number of benefits to AG-ACNPs, including the following:

1. Acknowledgment in One's Profession

Certification helps to build a practitioner's professional credibility and acknowledges their level of experience in their chosen sector.

It demonstrates the practitioner's dedication to preserving their clinical competence and serves as evidence of that commitment.

2. Moving Up in One's Profession

Achieving certification as an AG-ACNP might make it possible to enhance your career and take on leadership roles as well as enter specific practice areas.

Certified nurse practitioners are highly sought after or even required by many employers.

3. Improved Capability in Clinical Settings

The certification procedure encourages lifelong learning and ensures that AG-ACNPs are up to date on the most recent evidence-based techniques by requiring them to demonstrate such knowledge.

Certification places an emphasis on continuing education throughout one's career and a dedication to providing superior treatment to patients.

4. The Trust of Patients and Their Safety

Patients and their families have faith in certified practitioners since they are aware that these professionals have proven their level of expertise by meeting stringent requirements.

Certification demonstrates that the practitioner is committed to providing care of a high standard and level of safety.

An Overview of the Organizations That Offer the AG-ACNP Certification

Certification for the AG-ACNP can be obtained through one of two primary organizations:

The American Association of Critical-Care Nurses (AACN) comes in first place.

Through its Certification Corporation, the American Association of Critical-Care Nurses (AACN) presents the Adult-Gerontology Acute Care Nurse Practitioner Certification (AG-ACNP).

Because of its emphasis on acute and critical care, the AACN certification is widely recognized as being an excellent choice for individuals who are employed in medical facilities such as hospitals and intensive care units.

ANCC, which stands for the American Nurses Credentialing Center

The Adult-Gerontology Acute Care Nurse Practitioner-Board Certified credential is offered by the American Nurses Credentialing Center (ANCC).

The ANCC certification is applicable to a wide variety of practice settings, such as those for acute and critical care, primary care, and specialty care.

The Process of Obtaining the AG-ACNP Certification

The route toward obtaining the AG-ACNP certification consists of several important stages:

1. Requirements to Meet and Eligibility Requirements

The first thing you need to do is check to see if you are eligible to take the certification test that you want to take.

The normal requirements for eligibility include the possession of a valid and unrestricted registered nurse (RN) license as well as the successful completion of a graduate-level nursing program with an emphasis on adult-gerontology acute care.

Candidates should carefully evaluate the eligibility criteria of their preferred certifying organization in order to ensure that they meet the specific requirements, as these requirements may differ between the AACN and ANCC certifications.

2. The Application for the Exam

Candidates are required to send an application to the certifying organization once they have met the eligibility requirements.

The application process involves verifying the candidate's professional experience as well as their educational credentials.

The procedure for obtaining certification will typically involve payment of an application fee.

3. Studying for the Tests and Quizzes

The process of preparing for the certification exam is a substantial amount of work. Candidates will often devote a significant amount of time to studying in order to guarantee that they are sufficiently prepared.

Review classes, study materials, and practice tests are all beneficial components of an effective exam preparation strategy.

Candidates should also refer to the topic outline that has been provided by the certifying authority in order to direct their efforts toward studying for the exam.

4. An Examination for Certification

The certification exam represents the pinnacle of the process leading up to the certification. This test evaluates the candidate's knowledge and abilities in the areas of adult and geriatric acute care.

The candidate who is seeking certification from either the AACN or the ANCC will experience differences in the exam's structure, duration, and specific content.

In order for candidates to earn their certification, they are need to pass the exam.

5. Ongoing Certification Obligations

Once they have earned their certification, AG-ACNPs are required to take part in continuous certification maintenance activities in order to demonstrate that they are able to continue to fulfill the requirements of the applicable standards of practice.

Maintaining a certification often entails fulfilling requirements for further education and recertifying oneself on a periodic basis through testing or another method.

The Material Covered on the AG-ACNP Certification Exam

Examinations for the AG-ACNP certification include a wide variety of subject matter areas because the job requires a diverse set of knowledge and skills to perform well. The precise content areas that are tested on the AACN and ANCC exams could be slightly different from one another, but in general, they contain the following:

1. Evaluation and Clinical Diagnosis

Comprehensive patient evaluations, which include taking a medical history, doing physical exams, and interpreting diagnostic test results.

Clinical decision-making and differential diagnosis are also involved.

2. The most recent developments in clinical management

creating treatment plans for patients who have complex, acute, or critical health issues and then putting those plans into action.

pharmacological management, which includes the delivery of medications as well as the monitoring of their effects, both therapeutic and unfavorable.

3. The Promotion of Health and the Prevention of Disease

Methods to improve overall health, forestall disease, and control the symptoms of chronic health disorders.

Education and counseling of the patient regarding the avoidance of disease and the upkeep of their health.

4. Problems with Morality and the Law

Guidelines for ethical conduct and professional standards of practice for nurse practitioners.

Regarding the AG-ACNP's role, there are a number of legal and regulatory considerations.

5. Health Care Organizations and Public Policy

A comprehension of healthcare delivery models, healthcare policies, and healthcare delivery systems.

advocacy on behalf of patients as well as engagement in activities aimed at quality improvement and patient safety.

Hints and Guidelines for Your Preparation of the Certification Exam

1. Get a Head Start

Start working on your certification a significant amount of time before the exam that you want to take. The preparation for the test requires a significant investment of both time and effort.

2. Make Sure You Use the Appropriate Resources

Make sure that the study materials, review courses, and practice examinations that you use come from reliable sources. Make sure that they are consistent with the content outline that was provided by the organization that certifies people.

3. Construct a Learning Strategy

Create an organized learning plan for yourself that will cover all of the necessary content areas. Make sure that you give each subject the appropriate amount of time, and establish study objectives that are attainable.

4. Engage in Regular Practicing

You should evaluate both your knowledge and your ability to perform well on tests by using practice exams and questions. Get comfortable with the structure and flow of the certification test that you will be taking.

5. Seek Out Assistance

Think about being a part of a study group or making connections with other people in your field who are working toward the same certification. Motivation and additional learning materials are two things that can be provided by peer help.

6. Recreate the Conditions of the Exam

When you are practicing, try to recreate the conditions of the exam as accurately as you can. Set a timer for yourself, be sure to take pauses, and concentrate on questions similar to those on the exam.

7. Analyze the Weak Points

Determine which of your skills need more work, and focus your efforts there. It is vital to conduct a comprehensive review in order to overcome knowledge gaps.

8. Care for Oneself

Make taking care of yourself a top priority if you want to keep a good work-study-life balance. A mind that has been well-rested and is in a state of equilibrium is better able to take in and remember information.

9. Keep Yourself Informed

Maintain a state of current awareness on the most up-to-date clinical guidelines, research, and practice standards. The medical industry is always moving forward and becoming more advanced.

The Procedure for Ongoing Certification Maintenance

Following the completion of the AG-ACNP certification program, the next step in the path is certification maintenance:

1. Education That Never Stops

In order to keep their certification current, certified nurse practitioners are required by the majority of certifying bodies to complete a predetermined amount of continuing education credits.

It is important for AG-ACNPs to participate in ongoing education and to keep up with the latest developments in clinical guidelines, research, and best practices.

2. The re-certification process

Some organizations that grant certification mandate periodic recertification, which may take the form of an exam or another method. There are a few different approaches to the recertification procedure.

In order for candidates to keep their certification in good standing, the certifying organization they belong to has standards for recertification that must be met.

3. Code of Professional Conduct

Participation in professional activities on a regular basis is required. Clinical practice is where AG-ACNPs should demonstrate a consistent application of their knowledge and skills.

In professional practice, the utmost importance is placed on clinical skill, ethical behavior, and the protection of patients.

Gerontological care in adult-geriatric acute care nursing practice is covered in Chapter 12 of this book.

Adult-Gerontology Acute Care Nurse Practitioners (AG-ACNPs) are licensed healthcare professionals who specialize in providing acute care to older adults. One of their primary areas of focus is gerontological care. This chapter dives into the specific challenges that arise while providing medical attention to elderly patients in acute care settings. Particular attention is paid to the physiological, psychological, and social factors that must be taken into account in order to deliver all-encompassing and patient-centered care to this population.

A Brief Introduction to Geriatric Healthcare

Gerontology is a multidisciplinary field that focuses on the study of the aging process as well as the opportunities and difficulties that come along with it. The goal of gerontological care is to improve the health and quality of life of older people by concentrating on the physiological, psychological, and social components of the natural process of growing older.

AG-ACNPs are extremely important members of the gerontological care team because they provide advanced nursing treatment to elderly patients who are hospitalized for serious illnesses or who have several chronic conditions. This care takes a number of different clinical, psychological, and ethical factors into account.

The Problem of an Aging Population

The world's population is getting older, which is contributing to a dramatic shift in demographics that is currently taking place. This transition is being caused by several significant trends, including the following:

1. A Higher Anticipated Length of Life

The improvements in healthcare and living situations that have occurred in recent years have contributed to higher life expectancies.

As a direct consequence of this, the number of people who are considered to be older adults is on the rise.

2. Members of the Generation of Baby Boomers

The baby boomer generation, which includes people born between 1946 and 1964, accounts for a sizeable share of the population that is getting older.

This generation is frequently linked to ever-evolving requirements and needs in terms of healthcare.

3. Ailments that are Associated with Getting Older

Chronic diseases, such as heart disease, diabetes, and high blood pressure, are more likely to affect people as they age and are more likely to be fatal.

Gerontological care places a significant emphasis on the treatment and management of these disorders.

A Discussion of the Physiological Aspects of Geriatric Care

The physiological changes that come with being older have a substantial impact on the treatment that older people get in acute care settings. The AG-ACNPs are required to have a thorough understanding of these changes and the implications that they have for clinical practice:

1. Alterations in the Cardiovascular System

Alterations in both the anatomy and function of the heart can be seen with advancing age. These alterations have the potential to bring about diseases such as heart failure, arrhythmias, and hypertension.

The AG-ACNPs have a responsibility to be proficient in the management of cardiovascular problems and the monitoring for indicators of heart failure exacerbations.

2. Alterations in Respiratory Function

The risk of respiratory disorders such as pneumonia and chronic obstructive pulmonary disease (also known as COPD) increases with age as a result of age-related changes in the respiratory system, such as decreasing lung flexibility.

It is imperative to recognize these illnesses at an early stage and treat them in an efficient manner.

3. Changes in the Musculoskeletal System

Changes that occur in bones and muscles as a natural part of aging, such as a reduction in bone density and muscle mass, can contribute to an increased risk of fractures and falls.

The management of musculoskeletal disorders and the prevention of falls are two of the most important aspects of gerontological care.

4. Alterations in the Gastrointestinal Tract

Constipation, diverticulitis, and gastroesophageal reflux disease (also known as GERD) are some of the disorders that can develop as a result of the effects of aging on the digestive system.

Concerns about gut health and nutrition must be addressed by AG-ACNPs when treating older patients.

5. Alterations in the Renal

Changes that occur in the kidneys as a result of aging can lead to a reduction in kidney function as well as an increased risk of chronic kidney disease.

Care consists of many components, two of which are the management of renal problems and the monitoring of pharmaceutical safety.

A Discussion on the Psychological Aspects of Geriatric Care

Changes in one's mental state and cognitive abilities are an essential part of gerontological care. The following are some changes that AG-ACNPs need to be aware of and incorporate into their practices:

1. Impairment of Cognitive Function

Alzheimer's disease and other forms of dementia are significant causes of concern among people of advanced age. Care, diagnosis, and management of dementia are essential areas of expertise for AG-ACNPs.

Delirium, a reversible acute cognitive impairment, is also common in acute care settings, and it requires rapid evaluation and management in order to be properly treated.

2. Problems Relating to Mental Health

Depression and anxiety are common experiences among people of senior age. Screening for mental health difficulties and providing relevant solutions should be the responsibility of AG-ACNPs.

Even though suicidal ideation doesn't happen very often, it's still a serious problem that needs prompt attention.

3. The Standard of Living

Decisions about quality of life, such as end-of-life care, advance directives, and palliative care can be especially difficult for elderly people to make.

The AG-ACNPs play a crucial part in enabling these conversations and making certain that the patient's choices are honored.

The Aspects of Society That Are Involved in Geriatric Care

Because of the significant impact that social factors have on the health and wellbeing of older adults, gerontological treatment must pay careful attention to these factors.

1. Assistance from others

It is critical for older persons to maintain their social relationships and support networks. The AG-ACNP should evaluate the social network of an older adult and determine how it may affect the care they receive.

Isolation from others and a lack of companionship are significant problems that can have a negative impact on health outcomes.

2. Assistance to the Caregiver

Numerous elderly people rely on unpaid carers, most of whom are family members. Burnout and stress among caregivers are issues that frequently arise.

It is the responsibility of AG-ACNPs to provide caregivers with support and resources and to take into account the caregivers' requirements while planning care.

3. Having a Cultural Awareness

When giving care to older persons hailing from a variety of cultural traditions, cultural competence is absolutely necessary. It is important for AG-ACNPs to be sensitive to the cultural beliefs, values, and practices of their patients.

It is possible to improve both patient-provider interactions and the outcomes of healthcare by paying attention to cultural components of care.

4. Care Near the End of Life

Care provided to patients at the end of their lives is an important aspect of gerontological care. AG-ACNPs are frequently involved in conversations revolving around topics such as advance care planning, hospice, and palliative care.

It is absolutely necessary to make certain that patients' wishes are honored and that they are treated with dignity at all times.

Gerontological Care With Regards to Ethical Considerations

Gerontological care places a significant emphasis on ethical considerations. The AG-ACNP has to manage difficult ethical challenges, such as the following:

1. Independence and Free and Voluntary Consent

It is of the utmost importance to respect the autonomy of older persons, particularly their freedom to make decisions regarding their own medical care.

AG-ACNPs have the responsibility of ensuring that patients have access to all of the information they need to give informed consent.

2. Beneficence and non-maleficence in behavior toward others

In gerontological care, the essential principles that must be adhered to are those of doing good (beneficence) and avoiding doing damage (non-maleficence).

AG-ACNPs are tasked with analyzing the potential advantages and disadvantages of various treatments, particularly in the setting of comorbid conditions and intricate care regimens.

3. Telling the Truth and Being Honest

Even when discussing sensitive matters with patients and their families, such as terminal disease or decisions regarding end-of-life care, AG-ACNPs are expected to be truthful and honest at all times.

The establishment of trust and the upkeep of open communication are both vital.

4. Righteousness

The equitable distribution of medical resources is an example of distributive justice. It is the responsibility of AG-ACNPs to advocate for equal access to care and make certain that older adults receive the treatments they require.

They should also address discrepancies in the provision of healthcare and the results of that provision.

Gerontological Care Faces a Number of Obstacles

Gerontological care comes with its fair share of obstacles, some of which include the following:

1. the use of multiple medications.

It is common practice for older persons to take many drugs, which increases the risk of drug interactions, side effects, and non-adherence.

The AG-ACNP is responsible for conducting a thorough medication regimen assessment and should consider deprescribing when the situation calls for it.

2. Impairment of Cognitive Function and Decision-Making

The process of providing informed consent and making decisions regarding treatment plans might be made more difficult by cognitive impairment.

When it is deemed appropriate, AG-ACNPs should involve members of the patient's family or designated decision-makers.

3. Changes in Levels of Care

Transitions in care, such as moves between acute care, rehabilitation, and long-term care facilities, can be difficult for seniors and other elderly patients.

During transitions, AG-ACNPs are responsible for ensuring that there is appropriate communication and care coordination.

4. Care Near the End of Life

It can be taxing on one's mental state to provide end-of-life care that is both compassionate and appropriate. The end-of-life care demands of patients and their families must be addressed by AG-ACNPs, and these professionals must have the skills necessary to do so.

5. Obstacles of a Legal and Ethical Nature

In gerontological care, problems of a legal and ethical nature, such as those pertaining to questions of capacity, guardianship, and advance care directives, may surface.

It is expected of AG-ACNPs to have a thorough comprehension of the pertinent legal and ethical standards.

Caregiving Standards Appropriate for Older Patients

AG-ACNPs are expected to adhere to the following best practices in order to deliver excellent gerontological care:

1. All-Encompassing Evaluation

Carry out exhaustive evaluations that take into account the physiological, psychological, and social facets of care.

Ensure a comprehensive evaluation of both the patient's medical history and their present state of health.

2. Collaboration between Different Professions

Collaborate with a team that consists of professionals from several fields, such as social workers, occupational therapists, and physical therapists.

A holistic approach to treatment can be ensured when there is effective teamwork.

3. Care that is Focused on the Patient

When arranging patient care, make sure to put the patient's choices and values first. When it's feasible, include patients in the decision-making process as much as possible.

Think about coming up with individualized goals for older persons that are centered on improving their quality of life and their functional outcomes.

4. Preparing for Future Medical Needs

Have conversations on advance care planning, including the filling out of advance directives, and other such activities.

Make sure that the patients' wishes for their end-of-life care are recorded and respected.

5. The Management of Pain

Pay close attention to the management of pain in elderly patients. Effective treatment of pain requires using methods supported by evidence.

When dealing with people who have cognitive impairment, pay extra close attention to the assessment and management of their suffering.

6. Preventing Trips and Falls

The risk of falls among older adults should be evaluated and fall prevention strategies used.

Take into account things like the negative effects of medications, any muscle weakness, and any potential risks posed by the environment.

7. Administration of Medications

Regularly reviewing patient medication schedules and looking for ways to reduce or eliminate unnecessary prescriptions is essential.

It is important to educate both patients and caregivers about how to properly handle medications.

8. Having a Cultural Awareness

Maintain a level of cultural competence in the provision of medical care by recognizing and appreciating the variety of practices, beliefs, and values that exist.

Stay away from preconceptions and generalizations.

The Function of the AG-ACNP Within the Field of Gerontology

In the field of gerontological care, AG-ACNPs play an important role:

1. The Diagnostic Process and Treatment

In acute care settings, AG-ACNPs are responsible for the diagnosis and management of a wide variety of medical disorders that affect older persons.

Their knowledge is extremely helpful in delivering care and therapy that is supported by evidence.

2. Administration of Medications

The function of the AG-ACNP includes medication management as one of its primary responsibilities. They prescribe, make adjustments to, and monitor patients' medicine in an effort to achieve the best possible health outcomes.

3. More Recent Methods of Operation

As part of the care that they provide for critically ill older persons, AG-ACNPs are able to conduct sophisticated operations such as placing central lines and managing mechanical ventilation, among other things.

4. Instruction and Psychological Advice

Patients and their families are provided with information regarding the various health conditions, treatment options, and preventative measures.
Support and counseling on a psychological level are frequently essential components of gerontological care.

5. Treatment and Care Coordination

Care coordination is the responsibility of AG-ACNPs, who work in a variety of healthcare settings. They make it easier to shift from acute care to rehabilitation to long-term care after patients have been hospitalized.

6. Making Decisions in an Ethical Manner

AG-ACNPs participate in ethical decision-making and work to ensure that care provided to older adults is consistent with the values and preferences of those patients.

7. Policy and Political Influence

They advocate for the healthcare requirements of older persons and push legislation that improve gerontological care as well as access to treatment.

8. Research and New Product Development

A significant number of AG-ACNPs are active in research, which helps to advance the field of gerontological care and contributes to the development of best practices.

Wound care and procedures in adult-geriatric acute care nursing practice are covered in detail in Chapter 13.

Care for wounds is an essential part of nursing practice, and it is of utmost importance in the domain of adult-geriatric acute care nurse practitioners (AG-ACNPs), to name just one of the subspecialties that fall under this umbrella. This chapter investigates the difficulties of wound care within the context of acute care settings, as well as the specific procedures and interventions that AG-ACNPs deploy to enhance wound healing and improve patient outcomes in older persons.

An Overview of Wound Care Procedures Utilized in AG-ACNP Practice

Wound care is a discipline that involves extensive knowledge, clinical expertise, and a strategy that is centered on the patient. This sector also demands multidisciplinary collaboration. Wound care is an essential component of AG-ACNPs' practices since they commonly come into contact with patients who are suffering from acute and chronic wounds in hospital and acute care settings.

Different kinds of wounds

Because there are many different kinds of wounds, AG-ACNPs need to be skilled in evaluating and treating all of the following types of wounds:

1. Wounds Caused by Surgery

Wounds that are the result of intrusive operations like surgery can range from being very straightforward to being extremely complicated.

These wounds need to be closely monitored by AG-ACNPs for any signs of infection, dehiscence, or evisceration.

2. Pressure Sores or Pressure Injuries (Pressure Ulcers)

Pressure ulcers are localized injuries to the skin and underlying tissue, and they are often caused by pressure or pressure in combination with shear forces. Shear forces can also contribute to the development of pressure ulcers.

Assessment and prevention at an early stage are essential, as it can be difficult for wounds of this nature to heal in older persons.

3. Ulcers of the foot caused by diabetes

Ulcers of the foot caused by diabetes are a major cause for concern in diabetics over the age of 60 since neuropathy and impaired circulation are two of the factors that lead to their development.

The AG-ACNP is responsible for addressing wound healing while also managing the diabetes that is the underlying condition.

4. Ulcers of the Venous and Arterial System

Ulcers in the venous system are frequently brought on by venous insufficiency, whereas arterial ulcers are frequently brought on by inadequate blood flow.

In order to devise effective treatment programs, AG-ACNPs are required to discriminate between the various forms of ulcers.

5. Wounds Caused by Trauma

Accidents, falls, or injuries of some other kind can all result in traumatic wounds. They might range from being mild to really difficult.

It is absolutely necessary to evaluate the cause of the damage and to make sure that the evaluation is thorough.

6. Burns and

Wounds that have been burned might be the consequence of contact with heat, chemicals, or electricity. The management strategy is determined by the burn's extent and depth.

In order to properly direct treatment decisions, AG-ACNPs need to appropriately diagnose burns.

7. Wounds that are Chronic and Do Not Heal

Some wounds fail to heal and turn into chronic conditions. These may be the outcome of underlying health issues or infections that have not been resolved.

In order to address these complex wounds, AG-ACNPs are required to utilize advanced wound care procedures.

The Procedures Involved in Healing a Wound

The process of wound healing is dynamic and highly regulated. It consists of multiple phases that overlap and build upon one another.

1. Maintaining blood coagulation levels

Hemostasis, also known as the development of a blood clot for the purpose of controlling bleeding, is the first step in the process.

AG-ACNPs are tasked with ensuring sufficient clot formation while also keeping an eye out for excessive bleeding.

2. A state of inflammation

During the inflammatory phase, immune cells will begin to infiltrate the affected area in an effort to eliminate debris and pathogens.

AG-ACNPs are responsible for monitoring patients for any signs of infection or inflammation and initiating any necessary treatments.

3. Spread of Nuclear Weapons

The proliferation phase is characterized by the formation of new tissue, blood vessels, and extracellular matrix.

The growth of granulation tissue is encouraged by AG-ACNPs, which also examine the site for indications of delayed healing.

4. Reconstruction

During the remodeling phase, the wound gradually becomes stronger as the collagen is rebuilt and rearranged.

The AG-ACNP will keep an eye out for severe scarring and will endeavor to optimize cosmetic and functional results.

Evaluation and Diagnosis in the Field of Wound Care

The first step in providing proper wound care is performing a comprehensive assessment. AG-ACNPs are required to collect extensive information in order to properly guide treatment decisions:

1. An In-Depth Examination of the Wound

Determine the wound's stage, as well as its location, size, and depth. It is the responsibility of AG-ACNPs to measure wounds and document any changes that occur over time.

Conduct an inspection to determine whether there is any undermining, tunneling, or sinus tracts.

2. The Appearance of a Wound Bed

Investigate the wound bed to determine the type of tissue present, its color, and whether or not necrosis, slough, or foreign material is present.

Find out whether or not there is granulation tissue and whether or not there is epithelialization.

3. Evaluation of the Wound Perimeter

Examine the area of the patient's skin that is surrounding the wound for any symptoms of maceration, excoriation, or dermatitis.

Conduct an examination of the integrity of the skin and make a record of any changes or possible issues.

4. Drainage from a Wound

Examine the amount of wound exudate, as well as its color, smell, and consistency.

To control the exudate coming from the wound, consider using wound dressings.

5. Evaluation of the Infection

Examine the wound for any indications of infection, such as redness, warmth, an increase in pain, purulent drainage, and systemic symptoms.

It is essential to diagnose and treat infections as soon as they are discovered.

6. The Root of the Problem

Determine the underlying reasons of wounds that do not heal, such as diabetes, venous insufficiency, or arterial insufficiency.

It is absolutely necessary for wound healing to address these underlying issues.

Classification of Wounds Based on Their Severity

It is vital to correctly classify wounds in order to choose the right therapy and track progress:

1. The National Pressure Ulcer Advisory Panel (NPUAP)

The National Pressure Ulcer Advisory Panel (NPUAP) has developed recommendations that define pressure ulcers from Stage I (non-blanchable erythema) all the way up to Stage IV (full-thickness tissue loss). Pressure ulcers are staged according to these guidelines.

The treatment planning process cannot proceed without accurate staging.

2. A Classification of Diabetes-Related Foot Ulcers

Ulcers on the diabetic foot are categorized according to their depth (using systems such as the Wagner classification) and whether or not they are infected.

The strategies and actions for wound care are informed by the classification.

3. Classification of Burns Using the Rule of Nines

Burns are categorized according to their depth (superficial, partial-thickness, or full-thickness), as well as their extent (the proportion of the affected body surface area).

The severity of the burns, both in terms of their breadth and depth, is the primary factor in determining the level of treatment necessary.

4. Classification of Ulcers Based on Venous and Arterial Origin

The location, size, and characteristics of the lesion are taken into consideration while classifying venous and arterial ulcers.

Correct classification helps guide treatment decisions and pinpoints the underlying causes of a condition.

Interventions for Wound Care (Wound Care)

The following are some of the measures that AG-ACNPs utilize to enhance wound healing and reduce complications:

1. Debridement of the Wound

The wound bed is cleaned by debridement, which eliminates necrotic tissue, slough, and any foreign material present.

Sharp debridement, autolytic debridement, enzymatic debridement, and mechanical debridement are all examples of techniques that can be used.

2. Cleaning of the Wounds

In order to properly clean the wound, the debris and excess exudate need to be removed while the surrounding healthy tissue is disrupted as little as possible.

It is essential to clean wounds using the appropriate products and procedures.

3. Measures to Prevent Infection

It is critical to detect and treat wound infections as soon as possible when they occur.

Antimicrobial drugs and antibiotics that are administered systemically might be recommended, and there are also steps taken to cut down on the bacterial burden.

4. Dressings and Other Topically Applied Medications

The characteristics of the wound, the exudate, and the clinical aims are taken into consideration when AG-ACNPs choose wound dressings and topical medications.

Hydrocolloids, foams, alginates, and antimicrobial dressings are all types of dressings that might be used.

5. Negative Pressure Wound Therapy (NPWT), often known as "Therapy"

The administration of subatmospheric pressure is a component of negative pressure wound therapy (NPWT), which aims to hasten wound healing, cut down on edema, and better manage exudate.

NPWT is an option for treating complex wounds for AG-ACNPs.

6. Treatment with Compression

Compression therapy is an essential component in the treatment of venous ulcers as well as the prevention of venous stasis.

AG-ACNPs determine which compression devices are most suited and check for any potential complications.

7. Relieving Pressure

When treating diabetic foot ulcers, offloading is absolutely necessary. AG-ACNPs are trained to offer advice on the most appropriate footwear and strategies for pressure redistribution.

8. Treatment with hyperbaric oxygen (also known as HBOT)

The hyperbaric oxygen therapy (HBOT) provides 100 percent oxygen at an enhanced atmospheric pressure, which speeds wound healing and lowers the risk of infection.

When it is medically necessary, AG-ACNPs may refer patients to have HBOT.

9. Surgical Procedures and Treatments

Surgical operations may be required to treat certain conditions. During treatments such as debridement, grafting, or closure, AG-ACNPs work in collaboration with surgeons.

10. Treatment of Aches and Pains

The treatment of wounds is often excruciating. The AG-ACNP evaluates and manages wound-related pain by utilizing both pharmacological and non-pharmacological treatment modalities.

Education for Both Patients and Caregivers

Education that is both effective and engaging is essential in wound care:

1. Personal Hygiene and Preventative Measures

It is important to educate both patients and caregivers on wound self-care, including how to change dressings, maintain hygiene, and prevent further complications.

Provide them with the knowledge to identify symptoms of infection or consequences.

2. Hydration and proper nutrition

It is essential for the healing process to have adequate nourishment and fluid intake. It would be helpful if you could provide some direction regarding the necessary fluid intake and food requirements.

3. Administration of Medications

Patients should be made aware of how to properly manage their medications, including antibiotics, analgesics, and any adverse effects.

Make sure patients take their meds as prescribed.

4. Helping Hands and Way of Life

Take into account the psychological and social components of wound care by providing patients with emotional support and encouraging them to lead healthy lifestyles.

Encourage a constructive mindset as well as engagement in the recovery process.
The Obstacles Facing Wound Care

The management of wounds can be difficult, and AG-ACNPs are required to overcome a variety of obstacles:

1. A Failure to Comply

The healing process of a wound can be slowed down if treatment suggestions are not followed. The AG-ACNPs are responsible for identifying obstacles to compliance and providing individualized help.

2. Ongoing Wounds and Injuries

Chronic wounds can have a variety of factors contributing to their development and are notoriously difficult to heal. It is vital to take a holistic approach.

3. Health Problems That Are Complicated

Wound healing may be impaired in elderly patients who have many conditions at the same time. While treating wounds, AG-ACNPs address the underlying problems that led to the injury.

4. Problems During the Operation

Wounds that have been surgically repaired have an increased risk of developing consequences, including infection, dehiscence, and evisceration. It is imperative that action be taken right now.

5. Ache from a Wound

Patients often report that the pain from their wounds is very upsetting. The AG-ACNP is responsible for implementing pain management measures while also addressing the underlying cause of the wound.

Recent Advances in the Treatment of Wounds

The treatment of wounds is continuously developing in tandem with developments in technology:

1. The Most Recent Dressings

Healing of wounds can be sped up by the application of innovative wound dressings such biologic dressings and growth factor dressings.

These innovative dressings are used by AG-ACNPs when it is clinically necessary.

2. Care for Telewounds

Telewound care enables AG-ACNPs to monitor wounds remotely, which enables them to provide early interventions while also eliminating the need for patients to visit the clinic in person.

3. Therapies Designed to Regenerate

New regenerative therapies, such as cell-based therapies and products built from tissue, show promise for boosting the body's natural ability to mend wounds.

There is a possibility that AG-ACNPs will have the opportunity to take part in clinical studies or to implement these treatments into their practices.

4. Printing in three dimensions

The technology of 3D printing allows for the creation of individualized wound dressings and skin substitutes. AG-ACNPs investigate these new developments in order to provide better wound care.

The management of pulmonary conditions in adult and geriatric patients receiving acute nursing care is covered in Chapter 14.

In acute care settings, the treatment of patients' respiratory systems is an essential component of patient care for both adult and geriatric patients. This chapter examines the intricacies of pulmonary disorders as well as the diverse role that Adult-Gerontology Acute Care Nurse Practitioners (AG-ACNPs) play in assessing, diagnosing, and managing these conditions in order to maximize the outcomes for patients.

An Introduction to the Management of Pulmonary Disorders

The respiratory system is essential to human life, and maintaining its health is critical to achieving optimal fitness levels across the board. AG-ACNPs play an important part in the management of pulmonary disorders and are useful in managing acute and chronic respiratory difficulties in adult and elderly patients. They serve a major function in the management of pulmonary conditions.

The Structure and Function of the Respiratory System Anatomy and Physiology

In order to effectively manage pulmonary conditions, having a strong grasp of the anatomy and physiology of the respiratory system is fundamental:

1. The Upper Part of the Respiratory Tract

The nasal cavity, oral cavity, pharynx, and larynx are all included in the upper respiratory system. The air that is breathed in is cleaned, humidified, and warmed by it.

2. the lower portion of the respiratory tract

The trachea, the bronchi, the bronchioles, and the alveoli are all components of the lower respiratory tract. It is accountable for the exchange of gases.

3. The Trading of Gases

In the alveoli, an exchange of oxygen (O_2) and carbon dioxide (CO_2) takes place. During this process, oxygen is absorbed by the blood while carbon dioxide is expelled into the airways.

4. Muscles of the Respiratory System

Primary respiratory muscles include the diaphragm as well as the intercostal muscles, which are involved in both inhalation and exhalation.

The ability of these muscles to maintain their strength and function can be impacted by aging.

Conditions of the Lungs That Are Common

A wide variety of pulmonary diseases, such as the following, are seen by AG-ACNPs.

1. Chronic Obstructive Pulmonary Disease (often referred to as COPD).

Chronic bronchitis and emphysema are both part of COPD, which is defined by a restriction in airflow and symptoms related to the respiratory system.

AG-ACNPs manage COPD patients by doing assessments, managing patients' medication, and educating patients.

2. bronchial asthma

The chronic inflammatory illness of the airways known as asthma can lead to temporary or permanent obstruction of the airways.

Patients are instructed by AG-ACNPs on the proper use of inhalers as well as the identification and avoidance of asthma triggers.

3. The pneumococcus

Pneumonia is an acute infection that affects the lower respiratory system. It manifests itself with fever, cough, and soreness in the chest.

AG-ACNPs diagnose and treat pneumonia, which most of the time requires treatment with antibiotics.

4. Pulmonary Embolism, also known as PE

A pulmonary embolism (PE) is a disorder that can be fatal if it is caused by a blood clot that becomes stuck in the pulmonary arteries. It makes breathing difficult and might cause discomfort in the chest.

The AG-ACNP is responsible for making a quick diagnosis of PE and beginning anticoagulation treatment.

5. Cancer of the Lungs

The majority of people who pass away from cancer do so from lung cancer. It frequently manifests itself as a cough, hemoptysis, and loss of weight.

Early diagnosis, the planning of treatment, and the management of symptoms are all areas in which AG-ACNPs are involved.

Idiopathic pulmonary fibrosis (IPF) comes in sixth place.

The term interstitial lung disease (ILD) refers to a collection of lung conditions that are characterized by scarring and fibrosis. It will cause your lung function to become impaired.

In order to control ILD and improve patients' quality of life, AG-ACNPs work in conjunction with pulmonologists.

7. Acute Respiratory Distress Syndrome (often referred to as ARDS)

The acute respiratory distress syndrome (ARDS) is a serious lung illness that is accompanied with sudden respiratory failure. Infection, trauma, or septic shock could all bring about this condition.

AG-ACNPs take part in the management of ARDS, which includes providing supportive care and mechanical breathing as necessary.

Evaluation and Analysis of the Situation

The importance of an accurate assessment and diagnosis cannot be overstated when it comes to pulmonary management:

1. A Brief Overview of Health

It is crucial to get a full health history, which should include information on the patient's smoking history, environmental exposures, and family history of lung illness.

The AG-ACNP is responsible for assessing the risk factors associated with pulmonary diseases.

2. An examination of the body

Identifying pulmonary problems requires a comprehensive physical exam that should include a focus on the patient's breathing rate, lung sounds, and chest examination.

AG-ACNPs are trained to recognize symptoms of respiratory distress, including the usage of auxiliary muscles and chest abnormalities.

3. Pulmonary Function Tests, Otherwise Known as PFTs

Lung function is evaluated by pulmonary function tests (PFTs), which may include spirometry and lung volume measures.

The diagnosis and subsequent treatment plan are based on the results.

4. Research Involving Imaging

Radiographs of the chest and computed tomography (CT) scans of the chest can offer visual insights into the disease of the lungs.

AG-ACNPs are responsible for image interpretation and work closely with radiologists.

5. An analysis of the arterial blood gases (ABG)

Blood oxygenation and carbon dioxide levels are measured by ABGs, which contribute to the evaluation of gas exchange and acid-base balance.

The findings of ABG tests are used as a guide for oxygen therapy and ventilation management by AG-ACNPs.

6. Tests Conducted in Laboratories

Infectious diseases and inflammatory lung disorders can be more accurately diagnosed with the help of laboratory testing such complete blood counts and inflammatory markers.

These tests are interpreted by AG-ACNPs in order to arrive at a diagnosis.

7. Examen de bronchoscopie

Bronchoscopy enables direct sight of the airways and the collection of samples that can be cultured and used for diagnosis.

AG-ACNPs have the ability to give pre- and post-procedure care, as well as assist in bronchoscopy operations.

Interventions for the Management of Pulmonary Conditions

AG-ACNPs utilize a wide variety of treatments in order to treat pulmonary diseases, including the following:

1. Administration of Medications

Medication is an essential component in the management of pulmonary conditions. Anticoagulants, bronchodilators, corticosteroids, and antibiotics are some of the most regularly recommended medications.

The AG-ACNP is responsible for ensuring that the appropriate medicine, dosage, and patient education are used.

2. Treatment with Oxygen

Patients who are diagnosed with hypoxemia can benefit from oxygen therapy. AG-ACNPs decide on the most effective way of oxygen supply and the suitable flow rate.

Monitoring the amount of oxygen in the blood is absolutely necessary in order to prevent hypoxia or oxygen poisoning.

3. Ventilation by Means of Machines

In cases of severe respiratory failure, mechanical ventilation is used to support gas exchange and lessen the amount of respiratory distress experienced.

When it comes to the management of ventilated patients, AG-ACNPs work in conjunction with respiratory therapists and intensivists.

4. Physiotherapy for the Chest

In order to assist in the clearing of the airways, chest physiotherapy utilizes a variety of techniques, including percussion, vibration, and postural drainage.

AG-ACNPs evaluate the necessity of these interventions as well as their effectiveness.

5. Respiratory Therapy and Exercise

Patients who suffer from chronic lung disorders can benefit from pulmonary rehabilitation programs by increasing their exercise tolerance and overall quality of life.

Patients who are eligible for these programs may be referred to them by AG-ACNPs.

6. Stopping the Habit of Smoking

Quitting smoking is one of the most important things you can do to prevent and treat lung illness. Educating patients about the dangers of smoking and providing support for efforts to quit are two of the primary responsibilities of AG-ACNPs.

7. Hospice and Palliative Care

Palliative care is provided to patients with severe or end-stage pulmonary illnesses to help manage their symptoms, address their psychological needs, and provide support for end-of-life planning.

Palliative care is actively provided by AG-ACNPs who are actively involved in the process.

Complications and Obstacles in the Management of Pulmonary Conditions

The management of pulmonary conditions is not without its difficulties:

1. Acute Exacerbations of the Condition

Patients who suffer from chronic lung disorders are at risk of developing acute exacerbations, which require rapid medical attention.

The training that AG-ACNPs get prepares them to properly manage these types of emergencies.

2. Multiple comorbidities

Comorbidities tend to cluster in older persons, making it more difficult to treat their respiratory conditions.

AG-ACNPs coordinate care across multiple medical specializations in order to meet the patients' comprehensive requirements.

3. Compliance with Prescribed Medication

It is not always easy to maintain proper drug compliance. AG-ACNPs implement ways to enhance adherence and reduce barriers in order to facilitate patient care.

4. Instruction of the Patient

Education of the patient in an efficient manner is vital. AG-ACNPs employ a wide variety of instructional strategies and resources in order to encourage self-management.

5. Morally Complicated Situations

It is possible for end-of-life decisions, mechanical ventilation, or even advanced care planning to present an ethical conundrum.

AG-ACNPs participate in ethical conversations and respect the patients' values as well as their autonomy.

Developments in Respiratory Care and Treatment

The management of pulmonary conditions continues to develop in tandem with advances in technology:

1. The use of telemedicine

Telemedicine allows for the remote monitoring of respiratory problems and the provision of prompt interventions, hence lowering the number of patients who need to be readmitted to the hospital.

2. Ventilation in the Home

Patients who are suffering from chronic respiratory failure are increasingly turning to home mechanical ventilation.

AG-ACNPs are responsible for ensuring that correct device maintenance and support is provided in the home.

3. The Use of Biological Treatments

In lung illnesses, biologic treatments can target specific inflammatory pathways, providing patients with access to more individualized therapy options.

There is a possibility that AG-ACNPs will have a role in the administration and monitoring of these treatments.

4. Procedures That Are Only Slightly Invasive

When treating severe asthma, minimally invasive methods like bronchial thermoplasty are being investigated as potential treatments.

During the post-procedure care process, AG-ACNPs work in collaboration with pulmonologists.

The interpretation of cardiac rhythms in adult and geriatric acute care nursing practice is covered in Chapter 15.

Interpreting cardiac rhythms is a critical ability for adult-geriatric acute care nurse practitioners (AG-ACNPs), also known as adult-geriatric acute care nurse practitioners, who practice in acute care settings. This chapter investigates the intricacies of cardiac rhythms, their importance in patient care, and the function of AG-ACNPs in evaluating and treating cardiac rhythm disorders to provide the best possible outcomes for patients.

An Introductory Look at the Interpretation of Cardiac Rhythms

The interpretation of cardiac rhythms is a crucial part of providing acute treatment to patients of all ages, including adults and elderly people. AG-ACNPs are required to have a complete awareness of both normal and aberrant cardiac rhythms in order to recognize problems that could be life-threatening, give prompt interventions, and interact with interprofessional teams for the purpose of providing optimal patient care.

The Structure and Function of the Human Heart

It is essential to one's ability to interpret cardiac rhythms to have a solid understanding of the anatomy and physiology of the heart.

1. The Chambers of the Heart

There are a total of four chambers in the heart, including two atriums and two ventricles.

The ventricles are filled with blood during the systole of the atrium, which is followed by the systole of the ventricle, which pumps blood to the lungs and the rest of the body.

2. The System for the Conduction of Electricity

The sinoatrial (SA) node, the atrioventricular (AV) node, the bundle of His fibers, and the Purkinje fibers are all components of the heart's electrical conduction system.

The SA node is responsible for producing the electrical impulses that start each heartbeat, which are then followed by coordinated conduction throughout the heart.

3. The placement of the ECG Leads

Leads for an electrocardiogram, often known as an ECG, are attached to various parts of the body in order to monitor the electrical activity of the heart.

The conventional electrocardiogram with 12 leads offers a wealth of information regarding the rhythm and electrical conduction of the heart.

Rhythms of the Heart That Are Typical

It is essential to have a solid grasp of normal heart rhythms in order to identify any abnormalities:

1. The Normal Sinus Rhythm, often known as NSR

NSR is characterized by consistent P waves and a heart rhythm that ranges from 60 to 100 beats per minute. It is thought to originate in the SA node.

It is an example of an electrical conduction system that is well-coordinated.

2. Rhythms of the Atrium

Atrial arrhythmias are responsible for the irregular P wave patterns that are seen in atrial rhythms such as atrial fibrillation (AF) and atrial flutter.

The AG-ACNP evaluates the ventricular response to atrial arrhythmias and manages the problems that are linked with this assessment.

3. Rhythms of the Ventricles

Arrhythmias that originate in the ventricles and pose a risk to a patient's life include ventricular tachycardia (VT) and ventricular fibrillation (VF), both of which are referred to as ventricular rhythms.

The AG-ACNPs are responsible for recognizing these rhythms and beginning prompt interventions, like as defibrillation, as necessary.

Typical Abnormalities of the Heart's Rhythm

In acute care settings, AG-ACNPs come across a spectrum of cardiac arrhythmias, including the following:

1. Atrial Fibrillation (often referred to as AF)

A irregular and rapid atrial contraction pattern, accompanied by an erratic ventricular response, is diagnostic of atrial fibrillation (AF).

The AG-ACNP evaluates the patient for the risk of stroke, manages the patient's anticoagulant treatment, and controls the patient's ventricular response.

2. Atrial Fibrillation

Atrial flutter is characterized by structured atrial contractions occurring at a rapid rate, most often in conjunction with a regular response from the ventricles.

The AG-ACNP assesses the ventricular response as well as the available treatment alternatives.

3. Supraventricular Tachycardia, also referred to as SVT

SVT refers to a collection of arrhythmias that begin above the ventricles and cause the heart to beat at an accelerated rate.

The AG-ACNPs are required to discern between the various forms of SVT and manage them appropriately.

4. Ventricular Tachycardia, also referred to as VT

The life-threatening arrhythmia known as VT is characterized by regular and fast contractions of the ventricles. Ischemia or structural heart disease could be the cause of this condition.

AG-ACNPs evaluate the patient's hemodynamic stability and take immediate action to halt the trend toward VF.

5. Atrial Fibrillation (also known as AF)

ventricular fibrillation (VF) is a disorganized and fast ventricular rhythm that results in cardiac arrest because there are no effective contractions.

The AG-ACNPs take part in advanced cardiac life support (ACLS) procedures, one of which is the delivery of defibrillation.

6. Bradycardiac condition

Bradycardias feature heart rates that are lower than sixty beats per minute and can be the result of anomalies in the conduction system.

AG-ACNPs are responsible for the evaluation of symptoms, the determination of whether or not intervention is necessary, and the management of bradycardias.

Evaluation of the Rhythms of the Heart

An accurate assessment of cardiac rhythms requires the following series of actions to be taken:

1. An electrocardiogram, often known as an ECG

The electrocardiogram (ECG) is the principal technique that is used to record heart rhythms. The ability to analyze electrocardiogram tracings and differentiate between normal and pathological rhythms is required by AG-ACNPs.

2. Analysis of the Rhythm Strip

It is normal practice, while conducting a focused assessment of the heart's rhythm, to separate a rhythm strip from a typical 12-lead electrocardiogram.

In-depth analysis can be performed by AG-ACNPs with the help of rhythm strips.

3. Identification of the Rhythm

It is essential to determine the origin of the rhythm (whether it be atrial, junctional, or ventricular) in order to decide which therapies are appropriate.

The P wave, the QRS complex, and the interaction between the two are all things that an AG-ACNP will think about.

4. How to Calculate Your Heart Rate

Calculating the patient's heart rate with precision is necessary in order to determine the clinical relevance of the rhythm.

When calculating a patient's heart rate, AG-ACNPs may use a variety of approaches, depending on the regularity of the rhythm.

5. Evaluation of Clinical Signs and Symptoms

Assessment of rhythm must always begin with the patient's symptoms, which may include chest discomfort, dyspnea, dizziness, and syncope.

When performing rhythm analysis, AG-ACNPs take into consideration the patient's presentation.

Telemetry and monitoring of the patient's heart

Monitoring and telemetry of the heart are both extremely important in the process of diagnosing and treating arrhythmias.

1. Monitoring of the Heart Rate Continually

Patients who are at a higher risk of arrhythmias, such as those who have just undergone surgery or who are already diagnosed with a heart condition, receive continuous cardiac monitoring.

AG-ACNPs are responsible for analyzing telemetry data, spotting any changes, and initiating any necessary measures.

2. Alarm-Related Exhaustion

Because of the large volume of monitor alerts, alarm fatigue is a problem in settings where patients receive medical care.

The AG-ACNPs are responsible for establishing guidelines for the management of alarms and for prioritizing alerts according to their clinical importance.

Treatments Available for Heart Rhythm Disorders

A variety of treatments are utilized in the therapy of cardiac arrhythmias, including the following:

1. Treatment Using Medications

Antiarrhythmics, beta-blockers, and calcium channel blockers are some examples of the types of medications that may be provided to patients in order to control arrhythmias.

AG-ACNPs are responsible for evaluating both the efficacy of medications and any potential side effects.

2. Cardioversion using Electric Current

Certain arrhythmias, such as atrial fibrillation (AF) and ventricular tachycardia (VT), can be converted to normal sinus rhythm with the use of electrical cardioversion.

AG-ACNPs are responsible for coordinating post-cardioversion care as well as the procedures involved in cardioversion.

3. Ablation Performed Via Catheter

Ablation with a catheter is a treatment that removes faulty electrical pathways in the heart that are the cause of arrhythmias.

When it comes to ablation procedures, AG-ACNPs work in conjunction with electrophysiologists.

4. Medical Gadgets That Are Implanted

In cases of bradycardia and high-risk arrhythmias, implanted devices such pacemakers and implantable cardioverter-defibrillators (ICDs) are used to treat the condition.

AG-ACNPs educate patients on how to manage their devices and check how the devices are functioning.

5. Therapy that Prevents Blood Clots

Anticoagulation medication is necessary for patients with atrial fibrillation who are at risk of having a stroke.

The AG-ACNP evaluates the patient's risk of having a stroke, begins anticoagulation treatment, and monitors for bleeding problems.

Interpreting cardiac rhythms can be difficult due to a number of factors.

The AG-ACNPs are required to overcome obstacles in the interpretation of cardiac rhythms:

1. Arrhythmias that are Complicated

Due to the complexity of certain arrhythmias, understanding their meanings might be difficult at times.

When seeking advise from an expert, AG-ACNPs consult with cardiac electrophysiologists.

2. Administration of Medications

Due to the fact that antiarrhythmic drugs could potentially cause proarrhythmia as well as other side effects, managing these medications requires regular monitoring.

AG-ACNPs provide patients with education on drug management and also monitor them for any adverse effects.

3. Capability for Quick Decision-Making

When dealing with potentially fatal arrhythmias like VF, making snap decisions is absolutely necessary. AG-ACNPs go through extensive training that teaches them to react quickly and begin ACLS protocols.

4. Instruction of the Patient

In order to effectively manage arrhythmia over the long term, patient education is absolutely necessary.

AG-ACNPs are responsible for ensuring that patients comprehend their disease, treatments, and any necessary changes to their lifestyle.

Recent Developments in the Management of Cardiac Rhythms

The field of cardiac rhythm management is continuously being shaped by advances in the field:

1. Monitoring from a Distance

The ability for AG-ACNPs to evaluate device function and patient status through remote monitoring of implantable devices frees them from the need to make regular in-person visits.

2. Pacemakers Made Without Lead

regular pacemakers can be replaced with leadless pacemakers, which are smaller and less invasive devices than regular pacemakers.

Patients who have leadless pacemakers may have an AG-ACNP involved in the evaluation and management of their condition.

3. Machine Learning and Artificial Intelligence (also known as AI)

Applications that use artificial intelligence and machine learning help in the early diagnosis of arrhythmias by evaluating large volumes of patient data.

In order to improve arrhythmia detection, AG-ACNPs work in conjunction with data analysts and AI professionals.

4. Testing of Genetic Material

Hereditary arrhythmia syndromes can be identified through genetic testing, which also contributes to tailored treatment and risk assessment.

In circumstances where inherited arrhythmias are suspected, AG-ACNPs may consider conducting genetic testing.

Advanced Practice Nursing Procedures in Adult-Gerontology Acute Care Nursing Practice is the topic of Chapter 16.

Adult-Gerontology Acute Care Nurse Practitioners (also known as AG-ACNPs) play an essential part in the delivery of comprehensive, patient-centered care in acute care settings, and advanced practice procedures are an essential part of that position. This chapter examines the various operations that AG-ACNPs do, the therapeutic value of those procedures, and the significance of maintaining both proficiency and safety in the workplace.

An Overview of the Most Recent and Most Advanced Practice Procedures

When it comes to evaluating, diagnosing, managing, and treating patients in acute care settings, advanced practice procedures involve a wide variety of different approaches that AG-ACNPs use. These operations call for an exceptionally high level of clinical expertise, as well as skill and critical thinking. In order to provide care that is both safe and effective for patients, AG-ACNPs are required to keep their knowledge and skills up to date.

Competence in the procedures

Competence in the appropriate procedures is absolutely necessary for AG-ACNPs:

Knowledge Base: An in-depth comprehension of the procedure, including its indications and contraindications, as well as its potential problems and evidence-based guidelines.

Technical proficiency refers to the ability to carry out a process correctly while maintaining a focus on the patient's well-being and safety.

Clinical judgment is the capacity to evaluate when a procedure is required, analyze findings, and make judgments based on those findings in an informed manner.

Care that is patient-centered means that an effort will be made to provide treatments that are congruent with the patient's values, preferences, and informed consent.

Procedures that are both Invasive and Non-Invasive

An extensive variety of invasive and non-invasive procedures can be carried out by an AG-ACNP. Some instances are as follows:

1. the procedure of venipuncture

The procedure known as venipuncture involves putting a needle into a vein in order to draw blood samples for analysis in a laboratory.

AG-ACNPs are responsible for collecting samples while ensuring correct technique and reducing patient discomfort as much as possible.

2. Puncture of the Arterial Wall

In order to get arterial blood for blood gas analysis or to test vascular function, arterial puncture is typically performed.

Arterial punctures are performed by AG-ACNPs, most frequently in intensive care settings, with the goal of reducing the risk of complications.

3. Insertion of a Central Venous Catheter (also known as a CVC)

The insertion of a central venous catheter (CVC) entails inserting a catheter into a big central vein for a variety of reasons, including the delivery of medication, monitoring of hemodynamics, and hemodialysis.

CVCs are inserted by AG-ACNPs while maintaining a sterile procedure and while monitoring the patient for any potential consequences, such as infections or pneumothorax.

4. a procedure called a thoracentesis

Thoracentesis is the process of removing pleural fluid or air from the chest cavity in order to treat pleural effusion, alleviate symptoms, or assist in the diagnostic process.

During a thoracentesis, AG-ACNPs make sure the patient is positioned correctly and manage any potential issues that may arise.

5. A lumbar puncture, often known as a spinal tap

A lumbar puncture is a procedure that includes extracting cerebrospinal fluid for diagnostic purposes by inserting a needle into the subarachnoid space of the spine.

When treating a variety of neurological diseases, AG-ACNPs do lumbar punctures while taking steps to avoid any potential consequences.

6. Closure of the Wounds and Suturing

Wounds, incisions, and lacerations are all types of cuts that can be closed with suturing. This takes a very specific methodology as well as an understanding of how wounds heal.

Suturing wounds and ensuring proper wound care and follow-up are two of the responsibilities of AG-ACNPs.

7. Procedures of Aspiration and Injection in the Joint

The procedure of joint aspiration involves the removal of synovial fluid from a joint for the purposes of diagnosis or treatment.

In addition, AG-ACNPs are capable of administering joint injections, which include placing drugs or other therapeutic agents directly within the joint area.

8. Care for a Tracheostomy Device

The administration and upkeep of a tracheostomy tube and stoma are both included in the scope of tracheostomy care.

The AG-ACNP ensures correct cleanliness, evaluates for problems, and educates patients as well as caregivers on how to properly care for patients with tracheostomies.

9. Perform a paracentesis

The removal of fluid from the peritoneal cavity is what happens during a paracentesis procedure, which is typically done to treat ascites or to help with the diagnostic process.

The AG-ACNP performs the paracentesis, addresses any difficulties that may arise, and then provides care following the treatment.

10. An aspiration and biopsy of the bone marrow

Diagnostic methods such as bone marrow aspiration and biopsy are utilized to evaluate patients with hematologic conditions.

These treatments are carried out by AG-ACNPs, who pay special attention to the patient's comfort and safety during the process.

Methods of the Future and Emergency Medical Care

In intensive care units, AG-ACNPs frequently carry out the following sophisticated procedures:

1. Insertion of an Endotracheal Tube

To protect the patient's airway and make it easier to provide mechanical ventilation, a procedure called endotracheal intubation involves inserting a tube into the trachea.

Intubation is performed by AG-ACNPs, and they also verify that the tube has been placed correctly in order to sustain respiratory function.

2. Insertion of the Chest Tube

When a patient has a condition such as pneumothorax or hemothorax, an insertion of a chest tube is performed so that air, fluid, or blood can be drained from the pleural area.

AG-ACNPs are responsible for the insertion of chest tubes, the management of drainage systems, and the evaluation of patient response.

3. Pacing of the Heart Through the Veins

For the treatment of bradycardias and heart blockages, a procedure called transvenous cardiac pacing involves inserting a temporary pacing wire into the heart.

AG-ACNPs are responsible for monitoring and managing temporary pacing as well as assessing the patient for problems.

4. The use of defibrillation and cardioversion.

The abnormal heart rhythms known as atrial fibrillation and ventricular fibrillation can be returned to a normal rhythm with the medical procedures known as cardioversion and defibrillation.

In life-threatening circumstances, AG-ACNPs are the ones who carry out these procedures.

5. Intubation in a Rapid Sequence (also Known as RSI)

Patients who are at danger of aspiration or airway compromise may benefit from RSI, which is a coordinated method to produce paralysis and intubation in a safe manner.

Critical care and emergency conditions call for the use of RSI by AG-ACNPs.

Imaging and Interpretation for Diagnostic Purposes

The following diagnostic imaging investigations are within the scope of practice for AG-ACNPs:

1. X-rays of the chest

X-rays of the chest can be used to diagnose respiratory and heart disorders, locate fractures, or evaluate the positioning of medical devices.

AG-ACNPs are responsible for the interpretation of chest X-rays for the purpose of clinical decision-making.

2. ultrasonography

The evaluation of vascular access, pleural effusions, and abdominal pathology can all benefit greatly from ultrasound imaging.

AG-ACNPs are qualified to carry out as well as interpret ultrasonography examinations.

3. the process of echocardiography

The ability of echocardiography to produce images of the anatomy and function of the heart in real time is a significant contribution to the diagnosis and treatment of cardiac diseases.

Echocardiograms can be interpreted by AG-ACNPs so that cardiac performance can be evaluated.

Control of Infections and Procedures to Ensure Their Safety

The prevention of infection and the safe performance of procedures are of the utmost importance:

Hand Hygiene: In order to stop the spread of infections, AG-ACNPs ensure that they practice correct hand hygiene both before and after treatments.

approach Stéril: In order to lower the patient's likelihood of contracting an infection, invasive operations require the use of a meticulously sterile approach.

Before beginning any procedure, an AG-ACNP will make sure to get the patient's or their legal representative's informed permission.

Patient Positioning: The correct positioning of the patient is vital to the effectiveness of the procedure as well as the patient's comfort.

problems: AG-ACNPs are constantly on the lookout for the possibility of problems and are prepared to act quickly in case any arise.

Education of Patients and Obtaining Their Consent Before Treatment

The education of the patient is essential:

Before getting a patient's consent to a procedure, an AG-ACNP must first confirm that the patient or the patient's representative understands the procedure, its purpose, any potential risks involved, and any available alternatives.

Patients receive education regarding pre-procedure preparations, such as whether or not they should fast, how their medications should be adjusted, and how they should care for themselves after the treatment.

Clear post-operation instructions, including any limits, signs of complications, and follow-up visits, will be supplied to the patient after the treatment has been completed.

Reis porting and Documentation of Events

It essential to have accurate documentation:

Notes on the Procedure Detailed notes on the procedure include indications, steps in the procedure, patient responses, and any complications.

Documentation of Informed Consent It is required, both legally and ethically, that documentation of informed consent be kept.

Evaluation of the Patient After the Procedure AG-ACNPs are responsible for documenting evaluations of patients after procedures, including vital signs, pain levels, and patient comfort.

Problems that Can Occur With More Advanced Procedures

When executing more complex treatments, AG-ACNPs must overcome a number of obstacles, including the following:

Anxiety in Patients It is possible for patients to develop anxiety or fear due to the upcoming surgery. Anxiety can be alleviated through the use of communication and other calming tactics by AG-ACNPs.

Patients who have complicated comorbidities or who have illnesses that are unstable require careful examination and planning.

Situations That Require Immediate Attention In the field of critical care, situations that require immediate attention involve prompt decision-making and collaboration with the interprofessional team.

Complications may arise as a result of the procedure itself, including but not limited to bleeding, infection, or allergic reactions. The AG-ACNPs are responsible for appropriately managing these problems.

developments in the most recent iteration of advanced practice procedures

The implementation of more complicated procedures is continually made easier by innovations such as:

Telemedicine: Telemedicine platforms enable advanced practice nurse practitioners (AG-ACNPs) to consult with medical professionals and remotely assist patients through procedures when it is feasible to do so.

Training Based on Simulation: Simulation-based training helps advanced practice nursing assistants (AG-ACNPs) hone their procedural abilities and remain current with the latest recommendations for best practices.

Imaging Technologies That Are State-Of-The-Art Complex medical procedures can benefit from imaging technologies that are currently state-of-the-art, such as intraoperative MRI or 3D printing.

Miniaturization: Miniaturized devices and tools allow for less invasive treatments and lessen patient discomfort. Miniaturization refers to the process of making something smaller.

Patient and Family Education in Adult-Gerontology Acute Care Nursing Practice is the Topic of Chapter 17 of this Book.

The Adult-Gerontology Acute Care Nurse Practitioner (AG-ACNP) practice places a significant emphasis on educating both patients and their families. This chapter delves into the critical role that education plays in acute care settings, the specific issues that need to be taken into account when working with adult and elderly populations, and the effective ways for enabling patients and their families to control their own health care.

An Overview of Education for Patients and Their Families

Education of both patients and their families is a dynamic and varied component of AG-ACNP practice in acute care settings. It is the process of providing patients and their families with the knowledge, abilities, and resources that will enable them to participate in their own self-care, make educated decisions regarding their healthcare, and achieve the best possible outcomes for their health. Education acts as a conduit between patients and their healthcare professionals, facilitating collaborative decision-making and improving the quality of care that is patient-centered.

The Importance of Providing Education to Patients and Their Families

Patient and family education carries a number of important advantages, including the following:

1. Self-determination

Patients who get education are better able to take an active role in their own care, which contributes to a heightened sense of control and autonomy.

Patients who are well-informed have a greater likelihood of following their treatment regimens and engaging in healthy habits.

2. Gains in Quality of Results

Patients who receive education have a greater chance of having positive health outcomes, fewer readmissions to hospitals, and better disease management.

They are more positioned to notice early symptoms of problems and respond effectively when they do so.

3. An Improved Overall Quality of Life

Education gives patients the ability to better comprehend their diseases and the treatment options available to them, which ultimately leads to an improvement in the patients' quality of life.

This can be especially essential in geriatric care, helping older persons to keep their independence while also improving their well-being.

4. Avoiding Potential Problems and Obstacles

Patients and their families benefit from education because it enables them to notice and avoid the occurrence of probable consequences.

This may be an essential component of care for adult and elderly patients who also have co-occurring conditions.

5. Making Communication Easier to Access

Education that is effective improves communication between patients, their families, and the healthcare providers who treat them.

This communication can be quite helpful in the coordination of care and transitions that take place in acute care settings.

Educational Obstacles Facing Patients and Their Families

Education of the patient and the family poses additional challenges:

1. Literacy in Health Care

Patients' varying levels of health literacy can have an effect on their capacity to comprehend and use the information they get from their healthcare providers.

AG-ACNPs are required to conduct health literacy tests and adapt educational programming accordingly.

2. Restricted Amount of Time

Due to time restrictions, education may be shallower and more superficial in acute care settings.

The AG-ACNP is responsible for effectively communicating vital information while also meeting the requirements of the patient and their family.

3. Considerations Relating to One's Age

When dealing with elderly patients, it is important to keep in mind that age-related variables, such as cognitive decline or sensory impairments, may impact the patients' capacity to take in new information.

Teaching methodologies should be adapted by AG-ACNPs in order to accommodate these various circumstances.

4. Having a Cultural Awareness

In order to render care that is respectful of the cultural ideas and values held by patients, it is essential to ensure cultural competence in educational settings.

AG-ACNPs have a responsibility to be sensitive to the cultural diversity and preferences of their patients.

The Education of the Patient and Their Families Process

The patient and family education process consists of numerous important components, including the following:

1. The evaluation

The first thing that needs to be done is an evaluation of the patient's and their family's educational needs. This evaluation should take into account the patient and their family's existing knowledge, as well as their preferred learning style and any obstacles to comprehension.

For the purpose of gathering this information, AG-ACNPs make use of assessment tools, health literacy screening, and communication skills.

2. Preparation

Following the completion of the assessment, a specialized education plan is prepared. This plan lays out the goals, objectives, content, and techniques for education, as well as the resources that are available.

The ability of the patient to learn as well as any cultural, age-related, or cognitive characteristics that may effect learning are taken into consideration by AG-ACNPs.

3. Putting It Into Practice

The actual imparting of education is an integral part of the implementation process. This can take place at the patient's bedside, in a specially designed education area, or via telehealth modalities.

A variety of instructional strategies, such as vocal instruction, written materials, visual aids, and interactive demonstrations, are utilized by AG-ACNPs.

4. The assessment

The usefulness of education can be determined through evaluation. The AG-ACNP evaluates the patient and their family to identify whether or not they have attained the learning goals and whether or not they are ready to utilize the acquired knowledge and skills.

It is essential to evaluate the learner's comprehension and provide feedback.

5. Records and documentation

The patient's medical record will contain accurate documentation of the educational efforts made because of documentation. It consists of the material that was discussed, how well the patient understood it, and any treatments or resources that were offered.

Maintaining care continuity and keeping the interprofessional team informed requires meticulous documentation.

Considerations Regarding Age as They Apply to Geriatric Education

The education of elderly patients necessitates the following unique considerations:

1. Alterations to the Mind

Memory, attentiveness, and one's capacity to process complicated information can all be negatively impacted by cognitive changes.

In order to emphasize crucial ideas, AG-ACNPs will frequently repeat themselves and utilize terminology that is simplified.

2. Impairments to the Senses

Impairments of the senses, such as hearing or vision loss, can have an effect on one's ability to communicate.

The AG-ACNPs provide accommodations for these limitations by providing aids like as hearing equipment or materials printed in a larger font size.

3. Administration of Medications

Multiple drugs might be manageable for older persons. Education encompasses correct medication administration, the possibility of adverse effects, and the significance of being compliant with prescription regimens.

4. Protection Against Falls

Geriatric education places a strong emphasis on fall prevention strategies. Balance exercises, home safety precautions, and wearing the appropriate footwear are some of the fall prevention tactics that AG-ACNPs educate their students on.

5. Treatment and Management of Chronic Diseases

Patients who are elderly frequently suffer from chronic diseases. In educational settings, the emphasis is placed on comprehending these diseases, detecting their symptoms, and successfully managing them.

Communication That Is Focused On The Patient

Patient and family education necessitates communication that is centered on the patient.

1. Engaging in attentive listening

Active listening is a skill that AG-ACNPs hone in order to comprehend the concerns and preferences of patients and their families.

Listening helps build trust between people and ensures that instruction is individualized to each person's need.

2. Questions That Are Left Open-Ended

Patients and their family are encouraged to express themselves and to articulate their understanding when open-ended inquiries are used.

These questions are utilized by AG-ACNPs in order to investigate problems and clarify information.

3. Speaking in Plain Language

Using language that is easily understood by patients and their families helps to simplify and make more understandable difficult medical information.

It is easier to understand something if you avoid using jargon and medical terms.

4. Teach-Back Methodical Approach

In the teach-back technique, patients are questioned about what they have learnt and then asked to express it using their own words.

It offers instant feedback on comprehension and makes it possible to ask questions and obtain clarification when necessary.

5. A Respect for One's Own Independence

The liberty of patients and their preferences should always be respected. Patients are included in the decision-making process and care planning by AG-ACNPs.

Partnerships in care can be built via respectful communication.

The Role of Technology in the Education of Patients and Their Families

The function that technology plays in the education of patients and their families is becoming increasingly significant.

1. Electronic Health Records, also abbreviated as "EHRs"

Electronic health records (EHRs) facilitate the documentation and accessibility of educational materials, giving patients and their families the opportunity to review information whenever it is most convenient for them.

EHRs are put to use by AG-ACNPs as a means of educational dissemination.

2. Telemedicine

Platforms that promote telehealth provide remote education and follow-up, which makes it simpler for patients to gain access to knowledge and get their questions answered.

The AG-ACNP is responsible for adapting education to the many different telehealth modes.

3. Applications for Mobile Devices

Mobile applications and websites that are related to healthcare can serve as extra resources for the education of patients.

Patients may receive recommendations for reputable applications and websites from AG-ACNPs.

Education that Focuses on Families

The concept of education that is centered on families acknowledges the significance of involving families in the learning process:

In the context of patient care and support, particularly geriatric care, members of the patient's family frequently play important roles.

The AG-ACNP interacts with the patient's family to ensure that the family is aware of the patient's condition, treatment plan, and the proper way to give care in the patient's home.

In education, addressing the concerns of families and offering emotional support are also included.

Collaboration Across Professions in the Field of Education

Collaborating across professional boundaries is vital for the education of patients and their families.

When it comes to providing complete education, AG-ACNPs work in conjunction with a variety of different healthcare professionals, including pharmacists, physical therapists, and social workers.

As a result of this teamwork, patients are guaranteed to receive an encompassing education that covers all facets of their care.

Educational Breakthroughs for Patients and Their Families

Education of patients and their families is being made easier by ongoing innovations.

1. Rehabilitation Using Electronic Means

By facilitating remote patient education and rehabilitation exercises, telerehabilitation helps patients on their path to recovery and overall wellness.

2. Applications for mobile health, or mHealth

Patients are better able to take control of their health by using mobile health applications that provide interactive and individualized instruction.

3. Virtual Reality (VR), also abbreviated

Platforms for virtual reality give educational experiences that are completely immersive, particularly in the fields of pain management and physical therapy.

4. Resources Available in Multiple Languages

The availability of education to a wide variety of patient populations can be ensured by using resources in multiple languages.

Quality Improvement and Patient Safety in Adult-Gerontology Acute Care Nursing Practice is the Topic of Chapter 18 in this Book.

Adult-Gerontology Acute Care Nurse Practitioner (AG-ACNP) practice incorporates both quality improvement (QI) and patient safety as essential aspects of their work. This chapter examines the significance of quality improvement and patient safety, as well as its impact on the outcomes of healthcare, and the role that AG-ACNPs play in leading initiatives to improve the quality of care and safety in acute settings.

Getting Started with Quality Assurance and the Protection of Patients

Enhancing patient safety and the quality of treatment being provided are essential components of contemporary medical practice. They involve making concerted attempts to consistently improve the level of treatment that patients receive while simultaneously reducing the likelihood that they will suffer any adverse effects. Within acute care settings, AG-ACNPs play a crucial position in both leading and participating in programs that aim to improve care processes, patient outcomes, and safety standards.

Importance of Quality Improvement and Maintaining a Safe Environment for Patients

Initiatives aimed at improving quality of service and ensuring patients' safety have a number of important repercussions for the healthcare industry.

1. Improved Outcomes for Individual Patients

The efforts put into quality improvement (QI) lead to better patient outcomes, such as lower death rates, fewer complications, and more effective disease management.

This is of utmost significance in geriatric care since older people frequently have a diverse range of medical requirements.

2. Minimizing Expenditures

Through the decrease of inefficiencies, readmissions, and problems, quality improvement that is done well can contribute to cost savings.

This is of utmost importance in a time when efforts are being made to cut costs associated with healthcare.

3. Observance of All Regulations

The regulatory regulations and accrediting standards that apply to healthcare facilities place a strong emphasis on quality improvement and patient safety.

Maintaining compliance is required in order to keep a license and/or an accreditation.

4. The Contentment of the Patients

Patients nowadays anticipate receiving care that is both of high quality and safe. The patient's level of satisfaction will increase if these expectations are met.

Patients who are pleased with their care and outcomes are more likely to take an active role in their treatment and to successfully manage their health.

5. Risk Avoidance and Management

The efforts that are put into patient safety assist lower the likelihood of medical errors as well as allegations of medical malpractice, which in turn mitigates the liability of healthcare institutions.

AG-ACNPs play an important role in locating possible dangers and devising solutions to eliminate them.

The Fundamentals of Quality Assurance and Enhancement

The enhancement of quality is guided by a number of fundamental principles:

1. Care that Is Focused On the Patient

The needs, preferences, and values of patients are put first in quality improvement projects.

AG-ACNPs include patients in the decision-making process regarding their care and solicit their comments to use as a basis for future enhancements.

2. Practice that is based on evidence

The quality improvement activities are guided by evidence-based recommendations and best practices.

AG-ACNPs incorporate the most recent scientific findings into patient care and actively promote the use of these findings in clinical settings.

3. Collaboration Amongst Professionals from Different Fields

The quality improvement process is a group effort that involves many people working in the medical field.

Improvements are implemented with the help of AG-ACNPs, who collaborate with physicians, nurses, pharmacists, and other members of the team.

4. Making Choices Based on Data

The gathering, examination, and interpretation of data are vital aspects of quality improvement.

AG-ACNPs make use of data to determine areas that could use improvement, monitor progress, and assess results.

5. Ongoing Observation and Analysis with Feedback

The quality improvement process is a continual endeavor that calls for ongoing monitoring and input.

AG-ACNPs evaluate the effectiveness of interventions on a regular basis and make necessary adjustments to the plans.

Initiatives for the Protection of Patients

Quality improvement programs must include patient safety measures.

1. The Security of Medications

Errors in medication are a serious cause for concern. Initiatives aimed at improving patient safety prioritize the elimination of drug mistakes by emphasizing the importance of precise prescribing, administration, and patient education.

2. Measures to Prevent Infection

The incidence of healthcare-associated infections (HAIs) can be decreased by using infection control procedures.

The AG-ACNPs serve an important part in the promotion of vaccination programs, appropriate hand cleanliness, and isolation procedures.

3. Protection Against Falls

Patient falls are a significant cause for concern when it comes to safety in acute care, particularly for senior patients.

Fall risk assessments, fall prevention methods, and education for patients and their families are all things that AG-ACNPs implement.

4. Protection Against Pressure Sores

Ulcers caused by pressure are complications that can be avoided. Through skin evaluations, repositioning, and the use of support surfaces, patient safety programs hope to reduce the likelihood of patients developing pressure ulcers.

5. The Practice of Safe Surgery

Before beginning the operation, standard operating procedures call for the verification of the patient's identity, the marking of the surgical site, and the implementation of time-out measures.

Preoperative risk evaluations and safety checklists are something that AG-ACNPs take part in.

The Importance of AG-ACNPs to Both the Promotion of Quality Care and the Maintenance of Patient Safety

In both quality improvement and patient safety, AG-ACNPs play a one-of-a-kind role:

1. Initiatives That Will Lead the Way

Within their respective practice contexts, AG-ACNPs frequently take the initiative to initiate and manage quality improvement and patient safety projects.

They work together with teams comprised of experts from a variety of fields to establish goals, formulate action plans, and assess results.

2. Expertise in the Clinical Setting

The clinical experience of AG-ACNPs is utilized to determine areas that could use some further development.

They are in an excellent position to evaluate the quality of care provided, identify patterns in the outcomes of patients, and formulate plans to improve care procedures.

3. Guiding Practice That Is Based On Evidence

AG-ACNPs are responsible for guiding the implementation of evidence-based practice by incorporating the most recent research findings and guidelines into the care that they provide.

They advocate for the utilization of interventions that are supported by evidence in order to improve patient care.

4. Instruction of the Patient

Education of the patient is an essential component of both quality improvement and patient safety. AG-ACNPs are responsible for educating both patients and their families about the need of participating in safety programs as well as safe care practices.

5. Analyzing the Data and Performing Performance Metrics

The AG-ACNPs monitor the effectiveness of quality improvement and patient safety actions through the use of performance indicators and data analysis.

They determine how successful interventions are and base their judgments on the collected data in order to obtain the best possible outcomes for patients.

6. The Promotion of a Safe Culture

The AG-ACNPs encourage open communication, the reporting of adverse events, and continual improvement, all of which contribute to the culture of safety that they cultivate.

When it comes to resolving safety concerns, they suggest using an approach that is collaborative and does not involve punishment.

Improvement Strategies, Instruments, and Procedures for Quality

Quality improvement projects typically make use of the following tools and approaches:

1. The Plan-Do-Study-Act Cycle (abbreviated as PDSA)

The PDSA cycle is a methodical approach to quality improvement. It entails designing an improvement, putting it into action, analyzing the results, and taking appropriate action based on what was discovered.

This cycle is utilized by AG-ACNPs in order to test modifications, evaluate the impact of those changes, and refine processes.

2. A Root Cause Analysis (often abbreviated as RCA)

The root cause analysis, also known as RCA, is a technique for determining the reasons behind undesirable events or mistakes.

AG-ACNPs are members of RCA teams that investigate accidents involving safety and devise ways to avoid such occurrences.

3. Analysis of the Failure Mode and Its Effects (FMEA)

The FMEA methodology is a preventative method of risk assessment. It does this by locating probable failure modes in processes and evaluating the consequences of those failure modes.

FMEA is utilized by AG-ACNPs in order to forecast potential mistakes and take preventative measures before they manifest.

4. The Six Sigma methodology

Six Sigma is a methodology that is driven by data that tries to reduce the amount of flaws and deviations that occur in operations.

The ideas of Six Sigma may be utilized by AG-ACNPs in order to enhance both the procedures involved in patient care and the results obtained.

Patient Safety Organizations (also abbreviated as PSOs)

Organizations dedicated to patient safety play an important part in the overall effort to improve patient safety:

1. The Gathering and Examination of Data

PSOs are responsible for the collection of data on patient safety events, as well as the analysis of trends and the dissemination of information to healthcare practitioners.

AG-ACNPs draw upon the information provided by PSOs in order to inform safety actions.

2. the dissemination of best practices

PSOs are responsible for disseminating patient safety recommendations and the most effective procedures.

The provision of care by AG-ACNPs includes the implementation of these principles.

3. Various Methods of Reporting

PSOs provide reporting tools for healthcare personnel to utilize in order to communicate any issues or incidents pertaining to patient safety.

AG-ACNPs encourage reporting and actively participate in the resolution of concerns that have been reported.

Improvements in Patient Safety and Quality of Care Delivered to the Elderly

In the treatment of elderly patients, quality improvement and patient safety measures are of utmost significance:

1. Detailed Analyses of the Situation

AG-ACNPs are responsible for conducting in-depth assessments in order to identify potential weaknesses in elderly patients.

These assessments provide the foundation for individualized safety strategies and interventions.

2. The Reconciliation of Medications

In geriatric care, when multiple medications are frequently prescribed to patients, medication reconciliation is essential.

The AG-ACNP evaluates and updates patient prescription lists, educates patients about medication management, and works to minimize adverse drug reactions.

3. Risk and Vulnerability Assessments

Geriatric patients who are at risk for functional decline and falls can be identified through frailty exams.

Interventions that address frailty and lower the risk of falling are developed by AG-ACNPs.

4. Treatment and Prevention of Delirium

Delirium is a major cause for concern when it comes to the safety of elderly people. AG-ACNPs are responsible for putting delirium prevention methods into action, such as cognitive evaluations and early mobilization.

5. Involvement of One's Family

It is critical to the patients' well-being that their family be involved in their care at every stage. Families are informed about patient needs by AG-ACNPs, and they are included in decision-making regarding care.

Obstacles to Be Confronted in the Name of Quality Improvement and Patient Safety

The endeavors for quality improvement and patient safety are not without obstacles:

1. Opposition to New Experiences

When implementing new safety procedures or quality improvement efforts, encountering resistance to change is a regular occurrence.

The AG-ACNPs are responsible for engaging and motivating the healthcare teams to implement change.

2. Restricted Access to Resources

It is possible for quality improvement efforts to be hampered by resource limits such as time and financial constraints.

The AG-ACNPs have to come up with innovative solutions to resource problems and push for the appropriate support.

3. The accuracy of the data and the reporting of it

Accuracy in data collection and reporting are both necessary components of QI. Data that is inaccurate or incomplete can direct improvement efforts in the wrong direction.

AG-ACNPs are responsible for working to assure the quality of data and the reliability of reporting.

4. Aspects Related to Culture

The culture of safety and attitudes toward quality improvement can differ from one hospital facility to the next.

There is a possibility that AG-ACNPs will face opposition to safety initiatives owing to cultural issues.

Innovations for the Betterment of Quality and the Protection of Patients

Continued innovations continue to strengthen attempts to improve quality improvement and patient safety:

1. Analytical Methods in Healthcare

Innovative data-driven tools and analytics in the healthcare industry offer real-time insights into the quality of patient care and patient safety.

These tools are utilized by AG-ACNPs in order to keep track of trends and to respond in a proactive manner.

2. Artificial Intelligence, also referred to as AI

Applications of artificial intelligence assist in determining possible safety risks and predicting patient outcomes.

AG-ACNPs work together with data scientists to implement AI in a way that is safe for patients.

3. Standard Operating Procedures for Telehealth

Protocols for ensuring patients' safety while receiving care remotely are currently being developed in the field of telehealth.

The AG-ACNPs learn to adapt to these procedures in order to reduce the potential dangers involved with telehealth engagements.

4. Training in the Use of Interprofessional Simulation

Training in interprofessional simulation provides healthcare teams with the opportunity to practice safety and quality improvement initiatives in simulated environments that are true to life.

Simulation training is something that AG-ACNPs take part in to improve their teamwork and safety procedures.

Practice Questions and Answers Explanations 2023-2024

Question 1:
A 72-year-old patient presents with acute onset of chest pain, shortness of breath, and diaphoresis. An ECG reveals ST-segment elevation in leads II, III, and aVF. What is the most likely diagnosis?
A) Non-ST-segment elevation myocardial infarction (NSTEMI)
B) Atrial fibrillation
C) STEMI (ST-segment elevation myocardial infarction)
D) Unstable angina

Answer 1:
C) STEMI (ST-segment elevation myocardial infarction)

Explanation 1:
ST-segment elevation in multiple contiguous leads on an ECG is indicative of a STEMI. This patient should be urgently transferred to a catheterization lab for percutaneous coronary intervention (PCI).

Question 2:
Which of the following medications is commonly used to manage acute heart failure exacerbations in geriatric patients?
A) Angiotensin-converting enzyme (ACE) inhibitors
B) Beta-blockers
C) Loop diuretics
D) Calcium channel blockers

Answer 2:
C) Loop diuretics

Explanation 2:
Loop diuretics, such as furosemide, are often used to manage acute heart failure exacerbations in geriatric patients to reduce fluid overload.

Question 3:
A 65-year-old patient with a history of chronic obstructive pulmonary disease (COPD) presents with a productive cough, increased dyspnea, and fever. On auscultation, coarse crackles are heard. What condition should the AG-ACNP suspect?
A) Pneumothorax
B) Bronchitis
C) Pneumonia
D) Pulmonary embolism

Answer 3:
C) Pneumonia

Explanation 3:
The patient's symptoms of fever, productive cough, and coarse crackles on auscultation are suggestive of pneumonia, which can be common in patients with COPD.

Question 4:
In assessing an older adult's medication regimen, the AG-ACNP discovers that the patient is taking warfarin. Which laboratory test should be monitored to assess the patient's response to warfarin therapy?
A) Activated partial thromboplastin time (aPTT)
B) Prothrombin time (PT)
C) International normalized ratio (INR)
D) Platelet count

Answer 4:
C) International normalized ratio (INR)

Explanation 4:
The INR is used to monitor the patient's response to warfarin therapy. The target INR varies depending on the indication but is commonly maintained between 2.0 and 3.0 for most patients.

Question 5:
A 78-year-old patient is scheduled for elective surgery. The patient has a history of atrial fibrillation and is taking a direct oral anticoagulant (DOAC). What should the AG-ACNP recommend regarding the DOAC prior to surgery?
A) Continue the DOAC without interruption.
B) Stop the DOAC 12 hours before surgery.
C) Stop the DOAC 24 hours before surgery.
D) Stop the DOAC 48 hours before surgery.

Answer 5:
B) Stop the DOAC 12 hours before surgery.

Explanation 5:
In most cases, DOACs should be stopped approximately 12 hours before elective surgery to minimize the risk of bleeding during the procedure.

Question 6:
A 70-year-old patient is admitted with sepsis and acute respiratory distress syndrome (ARDS). What initial fluid resuscitation strategy should be employed for this patient?
A) Rapid administration of 1-2 liters of crystalloid fluid
B) Slow administration of 500 mL of crystalloid fluid
C) Rapid administration of 500 mL of colloid fluid
D) Slow administration of 1-2 liters of colloid fluid

Answer 6:
A) Rapid administration of 1-2 liters of crystalloid fluid

Explanation 6:
In sepsis, initial fluid resuscitation typically involves the rapid administration of 1-2 liters of crystalloid fluid to restore intravascular volume and improve hemodynamics.

Question 7:
A patient with advanced dementia is admitted with aspiration pneumonia. The patient is unable to communicate and lacks a healthcare proxy. What is the most appropriate ethical approach to care for this patient?
A) Aggressive measures, including intubation and mechanical ventilation
B) Comfort-focused care with antibiotics and oxygen therapy
C) Withdrawal of all medical interventions
D) Initiation of artificial nutrition and hydration

Answer 7:
B) Comfort-focused care with antibiotics and oxygen therapy

Explanation 7:
In patients with advanced dementia and a poor prognosis, comfort-focused care, which includes antibiotics for treatable conditions and oxygen therapy, is often the most ethically appropriate approach.

Question 8:
A 68-year-old patient with a history of atrial fibrillation is started on a direct oral anticoagulant (DOAC). Which laboratory test does not need to be routinely monitored for patients on DOAC therapy?
A) Complete blood count (CBC)
B) Prothrombin time (PT)
C) Activated partial thromboplastin time (aPTT)
D) International normalized ratio (INR)

Answer 8:
B) Prothrombin time (PT)

Explanation 8:
DOACs, unlike warfarin, do not require routine monitoring of PT or INR. Monitoring aPTT is also generally not necessary for DOACs.

Question 9:
Which assessment finding is suggestive of decompensated heart failure in an elderly patient?
A) Decreased jugular venous distention (JVD)
B) Increased urine output
C) Bilateral crackles on auscultation
D) Decreased blood pressure

Answer 9:
C) Bilateral crackles on auscultation

Explanation 9:
Bilateral crackles on auscultation are indicative of pulmonary congestion, a common finding in decompensated heart failure.

Question 10:
A 75-year-old patient is diagnosed with atrial fibrillation. The AG-ACNP is considering anticoagulation therapy. Which scoring system is commonly used to assess stroke risk in this patient and guide anticoagulation decisions?
A) CHADS$_2$ (Congestive heart failure, Hypertension, Age, Diabetes, Stroke)
B) Ranson's Criteria
C) Wells Criteria
D) Child-Pugh Score

Answer 10:
A) CHADS$_2$ (Congestive heart failure, Hypertension, Age, Diabetes, Stroke)

Explanation 10:
The CHADS$_2$ scoring system is commonly used to assess stroke risk in patients with atrial fibrillation and guide anticoagulation decisions.

Question 11:
A 70-year-old patient presents with abdominal pain, nausea, and vomiting. Physical examination reveals abdominal tenderness, guarding, and rebound tenderness in the right lower quadrant. What condition should the AG-ACNP suspect?
A) Gastroenteritis
B) Diverticulitis
C) Cholecystitis
D) Appendicitis

Answer 11:
D) Appendicitis

Explanation 11:
The patient's symptoms, along with abdominal tenderness, guarding, and rebound tenderness in the right lower quadrant, are suggestive of appendicitis.

Question 12:
Which of the following laboratory findings is indicative of disseminated intravascular coagulation (DIC) in a patient with sepsis?
A) Elevated platelet count
B) Prolonged prothrombin time (PT) and activated partial thromboplastin time (aPTT)
C) Decreased D-dimer levels
D) Normal fibrinogen levels

Answer 12:
B) Prolonged prothrombin time (PT) and activated partial thromboplastin time (aPTT)

Explanation 12:
DIC is characterized by a consumption of clotting factors, leading to prolonged PT and aPTT. It also typically results in decreased platelet count, increased D-dimer levels, and decreased fibrinogen levels.

Question 13:
A 65-year-old patient presents with sudden-onset confusion, weakness, and expressive aphasia. What type of stroke should the AG-ACNP suspect?
A) Ischemic stroke
B) Hemorrhagic stroke
C) Transient ischemic attack (TIA)
D) Migraine with aura

Answer 13:
A) Ischemic stroke

Explanation 13:
The patient's symptoms, including sudden-onset confusion, weakness, and expressive aphasia, are indicative of an ischemic stroke, commonly caused by a thrombus or embolism.

Question 14:
In a geriatric patient, which intervention is important to prevent hospital-acquired delirium?
A) Administering sedatives regularly
B) Encouraging sleep during the day
C) Providing hearing aids for all patients
D) Promoting early mobilization and orientation

Answer 14:
D) Promoting early mobilization and orientation

Explanation 14:
Early mobilization and orientation are important interventions to prevent hospital-acquired delirium in geriatric patients. Administering sedatives regularly can increase the risk of delirium.

Question 15:
Which medication is commonly used as a first-line treatment for atrial fibrillation to control the ventricular rate?
A) Warfarin
B) Aspirin
C) Metoprolol
D) Nitroglycerin

Answer 15:
C) Metoprolol

Explanation 15:
Metoprolol is commonly used as a first-line treatment to control the ventricular rate in atrial fibrillation.

Question 16:
A patient with acute respiratory distress syndrome (ARDS) is receiving mechanical ventilation. Which ventilator parameter is adjusted to reduce the risk of ventilator-associated pneumonia (VAP)?
A) Tidal volume
B) Respiratory rate
C) Positive end-expiratory pressure (PEEP)
D) Fraction of inspired oxygen (FiO2)

Answer 16:
C) Positive end-expiratory pressure (PEEP)

Explanation 16:
Adjusting the Positive End-Expiratory Pressure (PEEP) can help reduce the risk of ventilator-associated pneumonia (VAP) by maintaining alveolar recruitment and preventing lung collapse.

Question 17:
A 74-year-old patient is admitted with acute kidney injury. Which laboratory finding is suggestive of prerenal azotemia?
A) Elevated serum creatinine
B) Elevated urine output
C) Elevated fractional excretion of sodium (FENa)
D) Elevated urine sodium concentration

Answer 17:
C) Elevated fractional excretion of sodium (FENa)

Explanation 17:
Prerenal azotemia is associated with a decreased FENa (typically less than 1%) due to the kidneys conserving sodium in response to decreased perfusion.

Question 18:
A geriatric patient with heart failure is taking an angiotensin-converting enzyme (ACE) inhibitor. What potential side effect should the AG-ACNP monitor for in this patient?
A) Hyperkalemia
B) Hypertension
C) Hypoglycemia
D) Bradycardia

Answer 18:
A) Hyperkalemia

Explanation 18:
Hyperkalemia is a potential side effect of ACE inhibitors, as they can lead to increased potassium retention.

Question 19:
A patient with chronic obstructive pulmonary disease (COPD) is prescribed home oxygen therapy. The AG-ACNP should recommend which of the following oxygen delivery devices for long-term use?
A) Nasal cannula
B) Venturi mask
C) Simple face mask
D) Non-rebreather mask

Answer 19:
A) Nasal cannula

Explanation 19:
For long-term home oxygen therapy, the nasal cannula is often recommended for its comfort and ease of use.

Question 20:
A 70-year-old patient with a history of hypertension and type 2 diabetes presents with sudden-onset left-sided weakness and slurred speech. Which diagnostic test is most appropriate for evaluating this patient for an acute ischemic stroke?
A) MRI with diffusion-weighted imaging
B) Computed tomography (CT) without contrast
C) Cerebral angiography
D) Lumbar puncture

Answer 20:
A) MRI with diffusion-weighted imaging

Explanation 20:
MRI with diffusion-weighted imaging is the preferred diagnostic test for evaluating acute ischemic stroke, as it is highly sensitive for detecting early changes in brain tissue.

Question 21:
A 76-year-old patient with a history of hypertension and osteoarthritis is experiencing severe knee pain. Which non-pharmacological intervention should be recommended for pain management?
A) Opioid analgesics
B) Nonsteroidal anti-inflammatory drugs (NSAIDs)
C) Physical therapy and exercise
D) Topical capsaicin cream

Answer 21:
C) Physical therapy and exercise

Explanation 21:
Physical therapy and exercise are non-pharmacological interventions that can help manage knee pain, especially in older adults with osteoarthritis.

Question 22:
A 68-year-old patient presents with a severe headache, photophobia, and neck stiffness. What is the most appropriate initial diagnostic test to evaluate for a potential subarachnoid hemorrhage?
A) Computed tomography (CT) scan without contrast
B) Magnetic resonance imaging (MRI) of the brain
C) Lumbar puncture
D) Cerebral angiography

Answer 22:
A) Computed tomography (CT) scan without contrast

Explanation 22:
A non-contrast CT scan is the most appropriate initial test to evaluate for a subarachnoid hemorrhage, as it can rapidly detect blood in the subarachnoid space.

Question 23:
A 72-year-old patient presents with symptoms of dementia and progressive decline in cognitive function. Which assessment tool is commonly used to screen for cognitive impairment in this patient?
A) Glasgow Coma Scale (GCS)
B) Mini-Mental State Examination (MMSE)
C) Confusion Assessment Method (CAM)
D) Modified Rankin Scale (MRS)

Answer 23:
B) Mini-Mental State Examination (MMSE)

Explanation 23:
The Mini-Mental State Examination (MMSE) is a commonly used tool to screen for cognitive impairment and assess cognitive function in patients with dementia.

Question 24:
In a geriatric patient with chronic kidney disease (CKD), which dietary restriction is often recommended to manage electrolyte and mineral imbalances?
A) Low sodium diet
B) Low potassium diet
C) Low calcium diet
D) Low magnesium diet

Answer 24:
B) Low potassium diet

Explanation 24:
A low potassium diet is often recommended in patients with CKD to manage hyperkalemia, a common electrolyte imbalance in renal disease.

Question 25:
A 70-year-old patient with type 2 diabetes has uncontrolled blood glucose levels. Which class of medications is typically considered as the first-line treatment for uncontrolled type 2 diabetes in older adults?
A) Sulfonylureas
B) Biguanides
C) Dipeptidyl peptidase-4 (DPP-4) inhibitors
D) Sodium-glucose cotransporter-2 (SGLT-2) inhibitors

Answer 25:
D) Sodium-glucose cotransporter-2 (SGLT-2) inhibitors

Explanation 25:
SGLT-2 inhibitors are often considered as a first-line treatment for uncontrolled type 2 diabetes in older adults due to their glucose-lowering efficacy and cardiovascular benefits.

Question 26:
A geriatric patient is diagnosed with delirium. Which medication class is a common cause of delirium and should be assessed in this patient's medication regimen?
A) Benzodiazepines
B) Nonsteroidal anti-inflammatory drugs (NSAIDs)
C) Antipsychotic medications
D) Beta-blockers

Answer 26:
A) Benzodiazepines

Explanation 26:
Benzodiazepines are a common medication class known to cause delirium, especially in older adults. Evaluating the patient's medication regimen for potentially inappropriate drugs is crucial in managing delirium.

Question 27:
A 68-year-old patient is admitted with suspected myocardial infarction. Which cardiac enzyme is considered the most specific for myocardial injury?
A) Troponin I
B) Creatine kinase (CK)
C) Lactate dehydrogenase (LDH)
D) Aspartate aminotransferase (AST)

Answer 27:
A) Troponin I

Explanation 27:
Troponin I is the most specific cardiac enzyme for myocardial injury and is commonly used in diagnosing myocardial infarction.

Question 28:
A geriatric patient with a history of falls is at risk for osteoporosis. What imaging study is used to diagnose and assess bone density in osteoporosis?
A) MRI of the spine
B) Bone scan
C) Dual-energy X-ray absorptiometry (DXA) scan
D) Computed tomography (CT) scan of the pelvis

Answer 28:
C) Dual-energy X-ray absorptiometry (DXA) scan

Explanation 28:
A DXA scan is used to diagnose and assess bone density in osteoporosis, providing a T-score that quantifies bone density and fracture risk.

Question 29:
A 76-year-old patient is experiencing chronic pain from osteoarthritis. Which non-pharmacological intervention should the AG-ACNP recommend to manage this pain?
A) Opioid analgesics
B) Nonsteroidal anti-inflammatory drugs (NSAIDs)
C) Weight-bearing exercises
D) Hot and cold therapy

Answer 29:
C) Weight-bearing exercises

Explanation 29:
Weight-bearing exercises can help manage chronic pain from osteoarthritis by improving joint strength and function.

Question 30:
A 72-year-old patient with chronic kidney disease (CKD) is prescribed a phosphate binder. Which medication class is commonly used to manage hyperphosphatemia in CKD patients?
A) Loop diuretics
B) Calcium-based phosphate binders
C) Angiotensin-converting enzyme (ACE) inhibitors
D) Potassium-sparing diuretics

Answer 30:
B) Calcium-based phosphate binders

Explanation 30:
Calcium-based phosphate binders, such as calcium acetate and calcium carbonate, are commonly used to manage hyperphosphatemia in CKD patients by binding to dietary phosphate and reducing absorption.

Question 31:
A 70-year-old patient presents with persistent cough, wheezing, and dyspnea. On examination, inspiratory and expiratory wheezes are heard. What condition is most likely in this patient?
A) Pneumonia
B) Chronic obstructive pulmonary disease (COPD)
C) Pulmonary embolism
D) Asthma

Answer 31:
D) Asthma

Explanation 31:
The presence of wheezing, especially on both inspiration and expiration, is suggestive of asthma.

Question 32:
A geriatric patient is admitted with acute decompensated heart failure. Which class of medications is commonly used as a first-line treatment for reducing fluid overload and improving symptoms in this condition?
A) Thiazide diuretics
B) Aldosterone antagonists
C) Loop diuretics
D) Beta-blockers

Answer 32:
C) Loop diuretics

Explanation 32:
Loop diuretics, such as furosemide, are commonly used as first-line treatment for reducing fluid overload and improving symptoms in acute decompensated heart failure.

Question 33:
A 75-year-old patient is admitted with fever, cough, and purulent sputum production. Chest X-ray reveals consolidation in the left lower lobe. What is the most likely diagnosis?
A) Tuberculosis
B) Pneumonia
C) Pleural effusion

D) Lung cancer

Answer 33:
B) Pneumonia

Explanation 33:
The clinical presentation of fever, cough, purulent sputum production, and chest X-ray findings of consolidation are indicative of pneumonia.

Question 34:
In a geriatric patient with chronic kidney disease (CKD), which dietary restriction is commonly recommended to manage serum phosphorus levels?
A) Low sodium diet
B) Low potassium diet
C) Low phosphate diet
D) Low calcium diet

Answer 34:
C) Low phosphate diet

Explanation 34:
A low phosphate diet is often recommended to manage serum phosphorus levels in CKD patients.

Question 35:
A 72-year-old patient presents with generalized weakness, muscle cramps, and a positive Chvostek sign. What electrolyte disturbance should the AG-ACNP suspect in this patient?
A) Hypercalcemia
B) Hypokalemia
C) Hypernatremia
D) Hyponatremia

Answer 35:
B) Hypokalemia

Explanation 35:
The presence of generalized weakness, muscle cramps, and a positive Chvostek sign is indicative of hypokalemia.

Question 36:
A geriatric patient with atrial fibrillation is prescribed an anticoagulant for stroke prevention. What is the mechanism of action of direct oral anticoagulants (DOACs)?
A) Inhibition of platelet aggregation
B) Inhibition of vitamin K-dependent clotting factors
C) Direct thrombin inhibition
D) Promotion of fibrinolysis

Answer 36:
C) Direct thrombin inhibition

Explanation 36:
Direct oral anticoagulants (DOACs) work by directly inhibiting thrombin, a key component of the coagulation cascade.

Question 37:
A 70-year-old patient presents with acute chest pain that worsens with inspiration and improves when leaning forward. What condition is most likely in this patient?
A) Myocardial infarction
B) Pleurisy
C) Pneumonia
D) Gastroesophageal reflux disease (GERD)

Answer 37:
B) Pleurisy

Explanation 37:
The patient's chest pain that worsens with inspiration and improves when leaning forward is suggestive of pleurisy, which is often caused by inflammation of the pleura.

Question 38:
In an elderly patient, which laboratory value is commonly elevated in the setting of chronic inflammation or infection?
A) Hemoglobin
B) Serum albumin
C) C-reactive protein (CRP)
D) Glucose

Answer 38:
C) C-reactive protein (CRP)

Explanation 38:
C-reactive protein (CRP) is commonly elevated in the setting of chronic inflammation or infection and is a marker of acute-phase reactants.

Question 39:
A 75-year-old patient is admitted with a suspected gastrointestinal bleed. Which diagnostic test is most commonly used to localize the source of bleeding in the gastrointestinal tract?
A) Upper endoscopy
B) Magnetic resonance imaging (MRI)
C) Colonoscopy
D) Nuclear medicine bleeding scan

Answer 39:
A) Upper endoscopy

Explanation 39:
Upper endoscopy is commonly used to visualize and localize the source of bleeding in the upper gastrointestinal tract.

Question 40:
A 72-year-old patient with a history of congestive heart failure (CHF) presents with worsening peripheral edema and shortness of breath. On physical examination, jugular venous distention (JVD) is observed. What is the most likely diagnosis?
A) Acute pulmonary embolism
B) Pericardial tamponade
C) Decompensated heart failure
D) Cardiac tamponade

Answer 40:
D) Cardiac tamponade

Explanation 40:

The presence of JVD, peripheral edema, and shortness of breath is suggestive of cardiac tamponade, a condition where fluid accumulates in the pericardial sac and impairs cardiac function.

Question 41:

A 78-year-old patient with a history of hypertension and hyperlipidemia is prescribed statin therapy. What is the primary goal of statin therapy in this patient?
A) Lowering blood pressure
B) Improving glycemic control
C) Reducing serum cholesterol levels
D) Increasing hemoglobin levels

Answer 41:
C) Reducing serum cholesterol levels

Explanation 41:
The primary goal of statin therapy is to reduce serum cholesterol levels, specifically low-density lipoprotein (LDL) cholesterol, to decrease the risk of cardiovascular events.

Question 42:

A geriatric patient is diagnosed with dementia. What is the primary goal of treatment in managing dementia?
A) Curing the underlying cause of dementia
B) Slowing the progression of dementia
C) Managing behavioral symptoms
D) Reducing pain and discomfort

Answer 42:
B) Slowing the progression of dementia

Explanation 42:
The primary goal in managing dementia is to slow the progression of the disease, as there is currently no cure for most types of dementia.

Question 43:

A 74-year-old patient with a history of chronic obstructive pulmonary disease (COPD) presents with acute worsening of dyspnea, cough, and increased sputum production. What is the most appropriate initial treatment for this patient?

A) Intravenous antibiotics

B) Corticosteroids

C) Oxygen therapy

D) Beta-blockers

Answer 43:

B) Corticosteroids

Explanation 43:

In acute exacerbations of COPD, corticosteroids are commonly used as the initial treatment to reduce inflammation and improve lung function.

Question 44:

In a geriatric patient with heart failure, which class of medications is used to inhibit the renin-angiotensin-aldosterone system (RAAS) and reduce afterload?

A) Beta-blockers

B) Diuretics

C) Calcium channel blockers

D) Angiotensin-converting enzyme (ACE) inhibitors

Answer 44:

D) Angiotensin-converting enzyme (ACE) inhibitors

Explanation 44:

ACE inhibitors are used to inhibit the RAAS and reduce afterload in patients with heart failure.

Question 45:
A 70-year-old patient presents with sudden-onset chest pain and shortness of breath. ECG reveals ST-segment depression in multiple leads. What is the most likely diagnosis?
A) Non-ST-segment elevation myocardial infarction (NSTEMI)
B) Stable angina
C) Unstable angina
D) STEMI (ST-segment elevation myocardial infarction)

Answer 45:
C) Unstable angina

Explanation 45:
ST-segment depression on ECG is indicative of unstable angina, which is associated with ischemic symptoms at rest or with minimal exertion.

Question 46:
A geriatric patient is prescribed a new medication, and the AG-ACNP is concerned about potential drug interactions. Which resource can the AG-ACNP consult to assess potential drug-drug interactions?
A) The patient's family members
B) The healthcare organization's policy manual
C) A drug interaction database or software
D) The patient's primary care physician

Answer 46:
C) A drug interaction database or software

Explanation 46:
To assess potential drug-drug interactions, the AG-ACNP can consult a drug interaction database or software that provides information on medication interactions.

Question 47:
A 72-year-old patient presents with acute-onset chest pain radiating to the back. On physical examination, blood pressure is asymmetric, with lower pressure in the right arm compared to the left arm. What condition should the AG-ACNP suspect?
A) Myocardial infarction
B) Aortic dissection
C) Pulmonary embolism
D) Gastroesophageal reflux disease (GERD)

Answer 47:
B) Aortic dissection

Explanation 47:
The patient's acute chest pain radiating to the back, along with asymmetric blood pressure, is highly suggestive of aortic dissection.

Question 48:
In managing acute ischemic stroke, what is the primary goal of intravenous tissue plasminogen activator (tPA) administration?
A) Reducing intracranial pressure
B) Preventing seizures
C) Restoring blood flow to the ischemic brain tissue
D) Controlling hypertension

Answer 48:
C) Restoring blood flow to the ischemic brain tissue

Explanation 48:
The primary goal of intravenous tPA administration in acute ischemic stroke is to restore blood flow to the ischemic brain tissue.

Question 49:
A 70-year-old patient with a history of hypertension and diabetes presents with sudden-onset left-sided weakness and aphasia. What type of stroke should the AG-ACNP suspect?
A) Hemorrhagic stroke
B) Transient ischemic attack (TIA)
C) Ischemic stroke
D) Migraine without aura

Answer 49:
C) Ischemic stroke

Explanation 49:
The sudden-onset left-sided weakness and aphasia are indicative of an ischemic stroke, often caused by a thrombus or embolism.

Question 50:
A geriatric patient with a history of heart failure is prescribed an angiotensin-converting enzyme (ACE) inhibitor. Which potential side effect should be monitored in this patient?
A) Hypernatremia
B) Hypoglycemia
C) Hyperkalemia
D) Tachycardia

Answer 50:
C) Hyperkalemia

Explanation 50:
Hyperkalemia is a potential side effect of ACE inhibitors, as they can lead to increased potassium levels.

Question 51:
A 75-year-old patient with heart failure is prescribed an angiotensin receptor blocker (ARB). What is the primary mechanism of action of ARBs in the management of heart failure?
A) Reducing afterload
B) Increasing sodium retention
C) Inhibiting aldosterone release
D) Enhancing myocardial contractility

Answer 51:
A) Reducing afterload

Explanation 51:
The primary mechanism of action of ARBs in the management of heart failure is to reduce afterload by blocking the effects of angiotensin II on blood vessels.

Question 52:
A geriatric patient with a history of falls and gait instability is at risk for developing which neurological disorder?
A) Parkinson's disease
B) Alzheimer's disease
C) Multiple sclerosis
D) Huntington's disease

Answer 52:
A) Parkinson's disease

Explanation 52:
Gait instability and a history of falls are risk factors for the development of Parkinson's disease, a neurological disorder characterized by motor dysfunction.

Question 53:
A 72-year-old patient with a history of hypertension is taking a thiazide diuretic. What electrolyte disturbance should be monitored in this patient?
A) Hypernatremia
B) Hyperkalemia
C) Hypocalcemia
D) Hypokalemia

Answer 53:
D) Hypokalemia

Explanation 53:
Hypokalemia is a potential side effect of thiazide diuretics, which can lead to low potassium levels.

Question 54:
A 78-year-old patient with a history of chronic obstructive pulmonary disease (COPD) is admitted with acute exacerbation. What is the primary goal of oxygen therapy in this patient?
A) To raise oxygen saturation above 98%
B) To provide 100% oxygen via a non-rebreather mask
C) To relieve dyspnea and maintain oxygen saturation above 90%
D) To maintain oxygen saturation above 70%

Answer 54:
C) To relieve dyspnea and maintain oxygen saturation above 90%

Explanation 54:
The primary goal of oxygen therapy in a patient with acute exacerbation of COPD is to relieve dyspnea and maintain oxygen saturation above 90% while avoiding excessive oxygen to prevent hypercapnia.

Question 55:
A 70-year-old patient presents with sudden-onset confusion, lethargy, and difficulty speaking. On examination, the patient has right-sided hemiparesis and facial droop. What type of stroke should the AG-ACNP suspect?
A) Ischemic stroke
B) Hemorrhagic stroke
C) Transient ischemic attack (TIA)
D) Migraine with aura

Answer 55:
A) Ischemic stroke

Explanation 55:
The patient's sudden-onset confusion, right-sided hemiparesis, and facial droop are indicative of an ischemic stroke, which is commonly caused by thrombus or embolism.

Question 56:
A geriatric patient with a history of heart failure is prescribed a beta-blocker. What is the primary mechanism of action of beta-blockers in the management of heart failure?
A) Increasing heart rate
B) Enhancing myocardial contractility
C) Blocking the effects of catecholamines
D) Dilating blood vessels

Answer 56:
C) Blocking the effects of catecholamines

Explanation 56:

The primary mechanism of action of beta-blockers in the management of heart failure is to block the effects of catecholamines, reducing the workload of the heart.

Question 57:
A 72-year-old patient is admitted with severe chest pain that worsens with deep inspiration, tachycardia, and friction rub on auscultation. What condition should the AG-ACNP suspect?
A) Pneumothorax
B) Myocardial infarction
C) Pericarditis
D) Pleurisy

Answer 57:
C) Pericarditis

Explanation 57:
The patient's chest pain that worsens with deep inspiration, tachycardia, and friction rub on auscultation is indicative of pericarditis, inflammation of the pericardium.

Question 58:
A geriatric patient with chronic kidney disease (CKD) is prescribed an erythropoiesis-stimulating agent (ESA). What is the primary goal of ESA therapy in CKD patients?
A) Reducing serum phosphate levels
B) Enhancing bone mineral density
C) Improving hemoglobin levels and reducing anemia
D) Lowering blood pressure

Answer 58:
C) Improving hemoglobin levels and reducing anemia

Explanation 58:
The primary goal of ESA therapy in CKD patients is to improve hemoglobin levels and reduce anemia by stimulating red blood cell production.

Question 59:

A 74-year-old patient with a history of hypertension is prescribed an angiotensin receptor blocker (ARB). What is the primary mechanism of action of ARBs in blood pressure control?
A) Increasing cardiac output
B) Dilating blood vessels
C) Blocking the effects of aldosterone
D) Inhibiting platelet aggregation

Answer 59:
B) Dilating blood vessels

Explanation 59:
The primary mechanism of action of ARBs in blood pressure control is to dilate blood vessels, reducing systemic vascular resistance.

Question 60:

A geriatric patient with heart failure is prescribed digoxin. What parameter should be monitored when administering digoxin to avoid toxicity?
A) Blood glucose levels
B) Serum potassium levels
C) Serum creatinine levels
D) Serum digoxin levels

Answer 60:
D) Serum digoxin levels

Explanation 60:
When administering digoxin, it is important to monitor serum digoxin levels to avoid toxicity.

Question 61:
A 72-year-old patient presents with acute-onset chest pain, diaphoresis, and a feeling of impending doom. What is the most likely diagnosis?
A) Anxiety
B) Acute myocardial infarction (AMI)
C) Gastroesophageal reflux disease (GERD)
D) Pulmonary embolism

Answer 61:
B) Acute myocardial infarction (AMI)

Explanation 61:
The combination of acute-onset chest pain, diaphoresis, and a sense of impending doom is highly suggestive of an acute myocardial infarction (AMI).

Question 62:
A 70-year-old patient with chronic kidney disease (CKD) is prescribed a phosphate binder. Which dietary instruction should the AG-ACNP provide to this patient?
A) Increase dietary calcium intake
B) Limit dietary potassium intake
C) Restrict dietary protein intake
D) Avoid foods high in phosphorus

Answer 62:
D) Avoid foods high in phosphorus

Explanation 62:
Patients with CKD who are prescribed phosphate binders should be instructed to avoid foods high in phosphorus to reduce phosphorus intake.

Question 63:
A geriatric patient with a history of hypertension and heart failure presents with generalized weakness, fatigue, and cold intolerance. What thyroid disorder should the AG-ACNP suspect in this patient?
A) Hyperthyroidism
B) Hypothyroidism
C) Thyroiditis
D) Thyroid storm

Answer 63:
B) Hypothyroidism

Explanation 63:
The patient's symptoms of generalized weakness, fatigue, and cold intolerance are indicative of hypothyroidism, a condition where the thyroid gland does not produce enough thyroid hormones.

Question 64:
A 74-year-old patient is admitted with acute pancreatitis. What dietary intervention is recommended in the management of acute pancreatitis?
A) High-fat diet
B) Low-carbohydrate diet
C) NPO (nothing by mouth) status
D) Clear liquid diet

Answer 64:
C) NPO (nothing by mouth) status

Explanation 64:
In the management of acute pancreatitis, NPO (nothing by mouth) status is often recommended to rest the pancreas and minimize stimulation of pancreatic enzymes.

Question 65:
A 72-year-old patient with diabetes is prescribed an alpha-glucosidase inhibitor. What is the primary mechanism of action of alpha-glucosidase inhibitors in managing blood glucose levels?
A) Increasing insulin secretion
B) Enhancing glucose uptake by cells
C) Delaying carbohydrate digestion and absorption
D) Inhibiting gluconeogenesis

Answer 65:
C) Delaying carbohydrate digestion and absorption

Explanation 65:
The primary mechanism of action of alpha-glucosidase inhibitors is to delay the digestion and absorption of carbohydrates in the gut, resulting in slower increases in postprandial blood glucose levels.

Question 66:
A geriatric patient with heart failure is prescribed a diuretic. What is the primary goal of diuretic therapy in the management of heart failure?
A) Enhancing myocardial contractility
B) Reducing afterload
C) Improving cardiac output
D) Reducing fluid overload

Answer 66:
D) Reducing fluid overload

Explanation 66:
The primary goal of diuretic therapy in the management of heart failure is to reduce fluid overload by increasing the excretion of sodium and water.

Question 67:
A 70-year-old patient with a history of hypertension is prescribed a calcium channel blocker. What is the primary mechanism of action of calcium channel blockers in blood pressure control?
A) Reducing cardiac output
B) Blocking the effects of aldosterone
C) Dilating blood vessels
D) Increasing sodium retention

Answer 67:
C) Dilating blood vessels

Explanation 67:
The primary mechanism of action of calcium channel blockers in blood pressure control is to dilate blood vessels, reducing systemic vascular resistance.

Question 68:
A 76-year-old patient with heart failure is prescribed an angiotensin-converting enzyme (ACE) inhibitor. What is the primary mechanism of action of ACE inhibitors in the management of heart failure?
A) Reducing preload
B) Enhancing myocardial contractility
C) Inhibiting aldosterone release
D) Increasing afterload

Answer 68:
C) Inhibiting aldosterone release

Explanation 68:
The primary mechanism of action of ACE inhibitors in the management of heart failure is to inhibit the release of aldosterone, reducing sodium and water retention.

Question 69:
A geriatric patient with a history of falls and cognitive impairment is at risk for which type of fracture?
A) Hip fracture
B) Rib fracture
C) Clavicle fracture
D) Foot fracture

Answer 69:
A) Hip fracture

Explanation 69:
Elderly patients with a history of falls and cognitive impairment are at a higher risk of hip fractures, which can have significant morbidity and mortality.

Question 70:
A 72-year-old patient with chronic kidney disease (CKD) is prescribed erythropoiesis-stimulating agents (ESAs). What is the primary goal of ESA therapy in CKD patients?
A) Reducing serum phosphate levels
B) Improving hemoglobin levels and reducing anemia
C) Enhancing calcium metabolism
D) Lowering blood pressure

Answer 70:
B) Improving hemoglobin levels and reducing anemia

Explanation 70:
The primary goal of ESA therapy in CKD patients is to improve hemoglobin levels and reduce anemia by stimulating red blood cell production.

Question 71:
A 74-year-old patient is admitted with acute decompensated heart failure. What clinical finding is indicative of elevated central venous pressure (CVP)?
A) Hypotension
B) Elevated jugular venous distention (JVD)
C) Rapid weight loss
D) Decreased heart rate

Answer 71:
B) Elevated jugular venous distention (JVD)

Explanation 71:
Elevated jugular venous distention (JVD) is indicative of increased central venous pressure, a common finding in acute decompensated heart failure.

Question 72:
In a geriatric patient with atrial fibrillation, which class of medications is used for rhythm control by slowing atrioventricular (AV) conduction and restoring normal sinus rhythm?
A) Beta-blockers
B) Antiplatelet agents
C) Anticoagulants
D) Antiarrhythmic medications

Answer 72:
D) Antiarrhythmic medications

Explanation 72:
Antiarrhythmic medications are used to control rhythm by slowing AV conduction and restoring normal sinus rhythm in patients with atrial fibrillation.

Question 73:
A 70-year-old patient with a history of chronic kidney disease (CKD) is prescribed a loop diuretic. What electrolyte disturbance should be monitored in this patient?
A) Hypokalemia
B) Hyperkalemia
C) Hyponatremia
D) Hypocalcemia

Answer 73:
A) Hypokalemia

Explanation 73:
Hypokalemia is a potential side effect of loop diuretics, which can lead to low potassium levels.

Question 74:
A geriatric patient with heart failure is prescribed a beta-blocker. What is the primary goal of beta-blocker therapy in the management of heart failure?
A) Enhancing myocardial contractility
B) Reducing preload
C) Reducing afterload
D) Blocking the effects of catecholamines

Answer 74:
D) Blocking the effects of catecholamines

Explanation 74:
The primary goal of beta-blocker therapy in the management of heart failure is to block the effects of catecholamines, reducing the workload of the heart.

Question 75:
A 72-year-old patient with a history of heart failure is prescribed a thiazide diuretic. What is the primary mechanism of action of thiazide diuretics in the management of heart failure?
A) Enhancing renal sodium reabsorption
B) Reducing sodium and water retention
C) Increasing aldosterone release
D) Inhibiting catecholamines

Answer 75:
B) Reducing sodium and water retention

Explanation 75:
The primary mechanism of action of thiazide diuretics in the management of heart failure is to reduce sodium and water retention by inhibiting renal sodium reabsorption.

Question 76:
A geriatric patient with chronic kidney disease (CKD) is prescribed a potassium-sparing diuretic. What electrolyte disturbance should be monitored in this patient?
A) Hyperkalemia
B) Hyponatremia
C) Hypocalcemia
D) Hypokalemia

Answer 76:
A) Hyperkalemia

Explanation 76:
Hyperkalemia is a potential side effect of potassium-sparing diuretics, which can lead to elevated potassium levels.

Question 77:
A 70-year-old patient is admitted with acute shortness of breath, tachycardia, and wheezing. On examination, there is decreased breath sounds on one side and hyperresonance on percussion. What condition should the AG-ACNP suspect?
A) Pneumonia
B) Pleural effusion
C) Pneumothorax
D) Bronchitis

Answer 77:
C) Pneumothorax

Explanation 77:

The combination of decreased breath sounds on one side, hyperresonance on percussion, and acute shortness of breath is indicative of a pneumothorax, a condition where air accumulates in the pleural space.

Question 78:

A geriatric patient with a history of hypertension is prescribed an angiotensin receptor blocker (ARB). What is the primary mechanism of action of ARBs in blood pressure control?
A) Enhancing myocardial contractility
B) Inhibiting aldosterone release
C) Reducing cardiac output
D) Dilating blood vessels

Answer 78:

D) Dilating blood vessels

Explanation 78:

The primary mechanism of action of ARBs in blood pressure control is to dilate blood vessels, reducing systemic vascular resistance.

Question 79:

A 76-year-old patient with heart failure is prescribed digoxin. What parameter should be monitored when administering digoxin to avoid toxicity?
A) Blood pressure
B) Serum potassium levels
C) Serum creatinine levels
D) Serum digoxin levels

Answer 79:

D) Serum digoxin levels

Explanation 79:

When administering digoxin, it is important to monitor serum digoxin levels to avoid toxicity.

Question 80:

A 72-year-old patient with diabetes is prescribed an alpha-glucosidase inhibitor. What is the primary mechanism of action of alpha-glucosidase inhibitors in managing blood glucose levels?
A) Increasing insulin secretion
B) Enhancing glucose uptake by cells
C) Inhibiting gluconeogenesis
D) Delaying carbohydrate digestion and absorption

Answer 80:
D) Delaying carbohydrate digestion and absorption

Explanation 80:
The primary mechanism of action of alpha-glucosidase inhibitors is to delay the digestion and absorption of carbohydrates in the gut, resulting in slower increases in postprandial blood glucose levels.

Question 81:

A 78-year-old patient with a history of hypertension presents with sudden-onset chest pain, diaphoresis, and shortness of breath. On electrocardiogram (ECG), ST-segment elevation is observed in the anterior leads. What is the most likely diagnosis?
A) Non-ST-segment elevation myocardial infarction (NSTEMI)
B) Unstable angina
C) STEMI (ST-segment elevation myocardial infarction)
D) Stable angina

Answer 81:
C) STEMI (ST-segment elevation myocardial infarction)

Explanation 81:
The combination of sudden-onset chest pain, diaphoresis, and ST-segment elevation on ECG is highly suggestive of STEMI, indicating an acute myocardial infarction.

Question 82:
A geriatric patient with a history of diabetes presents with vision changes, including blurred vision and difficulty focusing. What complication of diabetes should the AG-ACNP suspect in this patient?
A) Diabetic retinopathy
B) Diabetic nephropathy
C) Diabetic neuropathy
D) Diabetic ketoacidosis

Answer 82:
A) Diabetic retinopathy

Explanation 82:
Vision changes, including blurred vision and difficulty focusing, are indicative of diabetic retinopathy, a common complication of diabetes affecting the eyes.

Question 83:
A 72-year-old patient with a history of heart failure is prescribed a loop diuretic. What is the primary mechanism of action of loop diuretics in the management of heart failure?
A) Increasing renal sodium reabsorption
B) Enhancing potassium reabsorption
C) Reducing sodium and water retention
D) Dilating blood vessels

Answer 83:
C) Reducing sodium and water retention

Explanation 83:
The primary mechanism of action of loop diuretics in the management of heart failure is to reduce sodium and water retention by inhibiting renal sodium reabsorption.

Question 84:
A geriatric patient with a history of atrial fibrillation is prescribed an anticoagulant. What is the primary goal of anticoagulant therapy in this patient?
A) Increasing platelet aggregation
B) Reducing the risk of thromboembolic events
C) Enhancing cardiac output

D) Controlling blood pressure

Answer 84:
B) Reducing the risk of thromboembolic events

Explanation 84:
The primary goal of anticoagulant therapy in a patient with atrial fibrillation is to reduce the risk of thromboembolic events, such as stroke.

Question 85:
A 74-year-old patient with a history of hypertension presents with acute-onset confusion, visual disturbances, and severe headache. On physical examination, blood pressure is significantly elevated. What is the most likely diagnosis?
A) Migraine with aura
B) Acute glaucoma
C) Hypertensive encephalopathy
D) Transient ischemic attack (TIA)

Answer 85:
C) Hypertensive encephalopathy

Explanation 85:
The acute-onset confusion, visual disturbances, severe headache, and significantly elevated blood pressure are suggestive of hypertensive encephalopathy, a severe complication of hypertension.

Question 86:
A geriatric patient with a history of chronic kidney disease (CKD) is prescribed an angiotensin-converting enzyme (ACE) inhibitor. What is the primary mechanism of action of ACE inhibitors in CKD patients?
A) Reducing serum cholesterol levels
B) Improving glycemic control
C) Reducing proteinuria and slowing the progression of CKD
D) Lowering blood pressure

Answer 86:
C) Reducing proteinuria and slowing the progression of CKD

Explanation 86:

In CKD patients, ACE inhibitors have a primary mechanism of action to reduce proteinuria and slow the progression of CKD.

Question 87:
A 70-year-old patient with a history of heart failure is admitted with acute decompensated heart failure. On auscultation, the AG-ACNP hears crackles at the lung bases. What does this finding suggest?
A) Pleural effusion
B) Pneumonia
C) Pulmonary edema
D) Pneumothorax

Answer 87:
C) Pulmonary edema

Explanation 87:
Crackles at the lung bases on auscultation are indicative of pulmonary edema, a common finding in acute decompensated heart failure.

Question 88:
A geriatric patient with a history of falls is at risk for which common musculoskeletal injury?
A) Achilles tendon rupture
B) Rotator cuff tear
C) Vertebral compression fracture
D) Meniscal tear

Answer 88:
C) Vertebral compression fracture

Explanation 88:
Elderly patients with a history of falls are at risk for vertebral compression fractures, which can lead to back pain and loss of height.

Question 89:
A 72-year-old patient is admitted with acute shortness of breath and chest pain. On physical examination, a friction rub is heard during auscultation. What condition should the AG-ACNP suspect?
A) Myocardial infarction
B) Pneumothorax
C) Pericarditis
D) Pleurisy

Answer 89:
C) Pericarditis

Explanation 89:
The presence of a friction rub on auscultation is indicative of pericarditis, an inflammation of the pericardium that can cause chest pain and shortness of breath.

Question 90:
A geriatric patient with heart failure is prescribed a beta-blocker. What is the primary goal of beta-blocker therapy in the management of heart failure?
A) Reducing preload
B) Enhancing myocardial contractility
C) Blocking the effects of catecholamines
D) Dilating blood vessels

Answer 90:
C) Blocking the effects of catecholamines

Explanation 90:
The primary goal of beta-blocker therapy in the management of heart failure is to block the effects of catecholamines, reducing the workload of the heart.

Question 91:
A 74-year-old patient is admitted with acute decompensated heart failure. On auscultation, the AG-ACNP hears a third heart sound (S3). What does the presence of an S3 sound suggest in this patient?
A) Aortic stenosis
B) Mitral regurgitation
C) Elevated left ventricular filling pressures
D) Ventricular tachycardia

Answer 91:
C) Elevated left ventricular filling pressures

Explanation 91:
The presence of an S3 heart sound suggests elevated left ventricular filling pressures, a common finding in acute decompensated heart failure.

Question 92:
A geriatric patient with a history of hypertension and hyperlipidemia is prescribed a statin. What is the primary goal of statin therapy in this patient?
A) Lowering blood pressure
B) Reducing blood glucose levels
C) Lowering cholesterol levels
D) Increasing platelet aggregation

Answer 92:
C) Lowering cholesterol levels

Explanation 92:
The primary goal of statin therapy in a patient with hypertension and hyperlipidemia is to lower cholesterol levels and reduce the risk of cardiovascular events.

Question 93:
A 70-year-old patient with a history of chronic kidney disease (CKD) is prescribed an angiotensin receptor blocker (ARB). What is the primary mechanism of action of ARBs in CKD patients?
A) Increasing serum creatinine levels
B) Enhancing renal sodium reabsorption
C) Dilating afferent arterioles
D) Reducing proteinuria and slowing the progression of CKD

Answer 93:
D) Reducing proteinuria and slowing the progression of CKD

Explanation 93:
In CKD patients, the primary mechanism of action of ARBs is to reduce proteinuria and slow the progression of CKD.

Question 94:
A geriatric patient with heart failure is prescribed an aldosterone antagonist. What is the primary mechanism of action of aldosterone antagonists in the management of heart failure?
A) Enhancing renal sodium reabsorption
B) Increasing potassium retention
C) Blocking the effects of angiotensin II
D) Reducing sodium and water retention

Answer 94:
B) Increasing potassium retention

Explanation 94:
The primary mechanism of action of aldosterone antagonists in the management of heart failure is to increase potassium retention while reducing sodium and water retention.

Question 95:
A 72-year-old patient with diabetes is prescribed metformin. What is the primary mechanism of action of metformin in managing blood glucose levels?
A) Increasing insulin secretion
B) Enhancing glucose uptake by cells
C) Reducing gluconeogenesis in the liver
D) Delaying carbohydrate digestion and absorption

Answer 95:
C) Reducing gluconeogenesis in the liver

Explanation 95:
The primary mechanism of action of metformin is to reduce gluconeogenesis in the liver, helping to lower blood glucose levels.

Question 96:
A geriatric patient with a history of heart failure is prescribed a calcium channel blocker. What is the primary mechanism of action of calcium channel blockers in the management of heart failure?
A) Enhancing myocardial contractility
B) Reducing afterload
C) Blocking the effects of catecholamines
D) Dilating blood vessels

Answer 96:
D) Dilating blood vessels

Explanation 96:
The primary mechanism of action of calcium channel blockers in the management of heart failure is to dilate blood vessels, reducing systemic vascular resistance.

Question 97:
A 70-year-old patient with a history of hypertension is prescribed a beta-blocker. What is the primary mechanism of action of beta-blockers in blood pressure control?
A) Increasing cardiac output
B) Dilating blood vessels
C) Reducing cardiac output
D) Blocking the effects of catecholamines

Answer 97:
D) Blocking the effects of catecholamines

Explanation 97:
The primary mechanism of action of beta-blockers in blood pressure control is to block the effects of catecholamines, reducing the workload of the heart.

Question 98:
A geriatric patient with heart failure is prescribed a thiazide diuretic. What is the primary mechanism of action of thiazide diuretics in the management of heart failure?
A) Enhancing renal sodium reabsorption
B) Reducing sodium and water retention
C) Increasing aldosterone release
D) Inhibiting catecholamines

Answer 98:
B) Reducing sodium and water retention

Explanation 98:

The primary mechanism of action of thiazide diuretics in the management of heart failure is to reduce sodium and water retention by inhibiting renal sodium reabsorption.

Question 99:
A 72-year-old patient with a history of heart failure is prescribed an aldosterone antagonist. What is the primary mechanism of action of aldosterone antagonists in the management of heart failure?
A) Reducing preload
B) Enhancing myocardial contractility
C) Inhibiting the release of aldosterone
D) Increasing afterload

Answer 99:
C) Inhibiting the release of aldosterone

Explanation 99:
The primary mechanism of action of aldosterone antagonists in the management of heart failure is to inhibit the release of aldosterone, reducing sodium and water retention.

Question 100:
A geriatric patient with a history of falls is at risk for which common musculoskeletal injury?
A) Achilles tendon rupture
B) Rotator cuff tear
C) Vertebral compression fracture
D) Meniscal tear

Answer 100:
C) Vertebral compression fracture

Explanation 100:
Elderly patients with a history of falls are at risk for vertebral compression fractures, which can lead to back pain and loss of height.

Question 101:
A 74-year-old patient with a history of hypertension presents with sudden-onset chest pain, diaphoresis, and shortness of breath. On electrocardiogram (ECG), there are no ST-segment changes. What is the most likely diagnosis?
A) Non-ST-segment elevation myocardial infarction (NSTEMI)
B) Unstable angina
C) STEMI (ST-segment elevation myocardial infarction)
D) Stable angina

Answer 101:
A) Non-ST-segment elevation myocardial infarction (NSTEMI)

Explanation 101:
The absence of ST-segment changes on ECG in a patient with sudden-onset chest pain, diaphoresis, and shortness of breath is indicative of NSTEMI.

Question 102:
A geriatric patient with a history of diabetes presents with symptoms of tingling and burning in the lower extremities. What complication of diabetes should the AG-ACNP suspect in this patient?
A) Diabetic retinopathy
B) Diabetic nephropathy
C) Diabetic neuropathy
D) Diabetic ketoacidosis

Answer 102:
C) Diabetic neuropathy

Explanation 102:
The symptoms of tingling and burning in the lower extremities are indicative of diabetic neuropathy, a common neurological complication of diabetes.

Question 103:
A 72-year-old patient with a history of heart failure is prescribed an angiotensin-converting enzyme (ACE) inhibitor. What is the primary mechanism of action of ACE inhibitors in the management of heart failure?
A) Reducing afterload
B) Enhancing myocardial contractility
C) Inhibiting aldosterone release

D) Increasing preload

Answer 103:
C) Inhibiting aldosterone release

Explanation 103:
The primary mechanism of action of ACE inhibitors in the management of heart failure is to inhibit the release of aldosterone, reducing sodium and water retention.

Question 104:
A geriatric patient with a history of atrial fibrillation is prescribed an anticoagulant. What is the primary goal of anticoagulant therapy in this patient?
A) Increasing platelet aggregation
B) Reducing the risk of thromboembolic events
C) Enhancing cardiac output
D) Controlling blood pressure

Answer 104:
B) Reducing the risk of thromboembolic events

Explanation 104:
The primary goal of anticoagulant therapy in a patient with atrial fibrillation is to reduce the risk of thromboembolic events, such as stroke.

Question 105:
A 74-year-old patient with a history of hypertension presents with acute-onset confusion, visual disturbances, and severe headache. On physical examination, blood pressure is significantly elevated. What is the most likely diagnosis?
A) Migraine with aura
B) Acute glaucoma
C) Hypertensive encephalopathy
D) Transient ischemic attack (TIA)

Answer 105:
C) Hypertensive encephalopathy

Explanation 105:

The combination of acute-onset confusion, visual disturbances, severe headache, and significantly elevated blood pressure is suggestive of hypertensive encephalopathy, a severe complication of hypertension.

Question 106:
A geriatric patient with a history of chronic kidney disease (CKD) is prescribed an angiotensin-converting enzyme (ACE) inhibitor. What is the primary mechanism of action of ACE inhibitors in CKD patients?
A) Reducing proteinuria and slowing the progression of CKD
B) Enhancing renal sodium reabsorption
C) Dilating afferent arterioles
D) Lowering blood pressure

Answer 106:
A) Reducing proteinuria and slowing the progression of CKD

Explanation 106:
In CKD patients, ACE inhibitors primarily reduce proteinuria and slow the progression of CKD.

Question 107:
A 70-year-old patient with a history of heart failure is admitted with acute decompensated heart failure. On auscultation, the AG-ACNP hears crackles at the lung bases. What does this finding suggest?
A) Pleural effusion
B) Pneumonia
C) Pulmonary edema
D) Pneumothorax

Answer 107:
C) Pulmonary edema

Explanation 107:
Crackles at the lung bases on auscultation are indicative of pulmonary edema, a common finding in acute decompensated heart failure.

Question 108:
A geriatric patient with a history of falls is at risk for which common musculoskeletal injury?
A) Achilles tendon rupture
B) Rotator cuff tear
C) Vertebral compression fracture
D) Meniscal tear

Answer 108:
C) Vertebral compression fracture

Explanation 108:
Elderly patients with a history of falls are at risk for vertebral compression fractures, which can lead to back pain and loss of height.

Question 109:
A 72-year-old patient is admitted with acute shortness of breath and chest pain. On physical examination, a friction rub is heard during auscultation. What condition should the AG-ACNP suspect?
A) Myocardial infarction
B) Pneumothorax
C) Pericarditis
D) Pleurisy

Answer 109:
C) Pericarditis

Explanation 109:
The presence of a friction rub on auscultation is indicative of pericarditis, an inflammation of the pericardium that can cause chest pain and shortness of breath.

Question 110:
A geriatric patient with heart failure is prescribed a beta-blocker. What is the primary goal of beta-blocker therapy in the management of heart failure?
A) Reducing preload
B) Enhancing myocardial contractility
C) Blocking the effects of catecholamines
D) Dilating blood vessels

Answer 110:
C) Blocking the effects of catecholamines

Explanation 110:
The primary goal of beta-blocker therapy in the management of heart failure is to block the effects of catecholamines, reducing the workload of the heart.

Question 111:
A 74-year-old patient is admitted with acute decompensated heart failure. On auscultation, the AG-ACNP hears a third heart sound (S3). What does the presence of an S3 sound suggest in this patient?
A) Aortic stenosis
B) Mitral regurgitation
C) Elevated left ventricular filling pressures
D) Ventricular tachycardia

Answer 111:
C) Elevated left ventricular filling pressures

Explanation 111:
The presence of an S3 heart sound suggests elevated left ventricular filling pressures, a common finding in acute decompensated heart failure.

Question 112:
A geriatric patient with a history of hypertension and hyperlipidemia is prescribed a statin. What is the primary goal of statin therapy in this patient?
A) Lowering blood pressure
B) Reducing blood glucose levels
C) Lowering cholesterol levels
D) Increasing platelet aggregation

Answer 112:
C) Lowering cholesterol levels

Explanation 112:
The primary goal of statin therapy in a patient with hypertension and hyperlipidemia is to lower cholesterol levels and reduce the risk of cardiovascular events.

Question 113:
A 70-year-old patient with a history of chronic kidney disease (CKD) is prescribed an angiotensin receptor blocker (ARB). What is the primary mechanism of action of ARBs in CKD patients?
A) Increasing serum creatinine levels
B) Enhancing renal sodium reabsorption
C) Dilating afferent arterioles
D) Reducing proteinuria and slowing the progression of CKD

Answer 113:
D) Reducing proteinuria and slowing the progression of CKD

Explanation 113:
In CKD patients, the primary mechanism of action of ARBs is to reduce proteinuria and slow the progression of CKD.

Question 114:
A geriatric patient with heart failure is prescribed an aldosterone antagonist. What is the primary mechanism of action of aldosterone antagonists in the management of heart failure?
A) Reducing preload
B) Enhancing myocardial contractility
C) Inhibiting the release of aldosterone
D) Increasing afterload

Answer 114:
C) Inhibiting the release of aldosterone

Explanation 114:
The primary mechanism of action of aldosterone antagonists in the management of heart failure is to inhibit the release of aldosterone, reducing sodium and water retention.

Question 115:
A geriatric patient with a history of falls is at risk for which common musculoskeletal injury?
A) Achilles tendon rupture
B) Rotator cuff tear
C) Vertebral compression fracture
D) Meniscal tear

Answer 115:
C) Vertebral compression fracture

Explanation 115:
Elderly patients with a history of falls are at risk for vertebral compression fractures, which can lead to back pain and loss of height.

Question 116:
A 74-year-old patient with a history of hypertension presents with sudden-onset chest pain, diaphoresis, and shortness of breath. On electrocardiogram (ECG), there are no ST-segment changes. What is the most likely diagnosis?
A) Non-ST-segment elevation myocardial infarction (NSTEMI)
B) Unstable angina
C) STEMI (ST-segment elevation myocardial infarction)
D) Stable angina

Answer 116:
B) Unstable angina

Explanation 116:
The absence of ST-segment changes on ECG in a patient with sudden-onset chest pain, diaphoresis, and shortness of breath is indicative of unstable angina.

Question 117:
A geriatric patient with a history of diabetes presents with symptoms of tingling and burning in the lower extremities. What complication of diabetes should the AG-ACNP suspect in this patient?
A) Diabetic retinopathy
B) Diabetic nephropathy
C) Diabetic neuropathy
D) Diabetic ketoacidosis

Answer 117:
C) Diabetic neuropathy

Explanation 117:

The symptoms of tingling and burning in the lower extremities are indicative of diabetic neuropathy, a common neurological complication of diabetes.

Question 118:

A 72-year-old patient with heart failure is prescribed an angiotensin-converting enzyme (ACE) inhibitor. What is the primary mechanism of action of ACE inhibitors in the management of heart failure?
A) Reducing preload
B) Enhancing myocardial contractility
C) Inhibiting aldosterone release
D) Increasing preload

Answer 118:
C) Inhibiting aldosterone release

Explanation 118:
The primary mechanism of action of ACE inhibitors in the management of heart failure is to inhibit the release of aldosterone, reducing sodium and water retention.

Question 119:

A geriatric patient with a history of atrial fibrillation is prescribed an anticoagulant. What is the primary goal of anticoagulant therapy in this patient?
A) Increasing platelet aggregation
B) Reducing the risk of thromboembolic events
C) Enhancing cardiac output
D) Controlling blood pressure

Answer 119:
B) Reducing the risk of thromboembolic events

Explanation 119:
The primary goal of anticoagulant therapy in a patient with atrial fibrillation is to reduce the risk of thromboembolic events, such as stroke.

Question 120:
A 74-year-old patient with a history of hypertension presents with sudden-onset chest pain, diaphoresis, and shortness of breath. On electrocardiogram (ECG), there are no ST-segment changes. What is the most likely diagnosis?
A) Migraine with aura
B) Acute glaucoma
C) Hypertensive encephalopathy
D) Transient ischemic attack (TIA)

Answer 120:
C) Hypertensive encephalopathy

Explanation 120:
The combination of sudden-onset chest pain, diaphoresis, and no ST-segment changes on ECG is suggestive of hypertensive encephalopathy, a severe complication of hypertension.

Question 121:
A geriatric patient with a history of chronic kidney disease (CKD) is prescribed an angiotensin-converting enzyme (ACE) inhibitor. What is the primary mechanism of action of ACE inhibitors in CKD patients?
A) Reducing proteinuria and slowing the progression of CKD
B) Enhancing renal sodium reabsorption
C) Dilating afferent arterioles
D) Lowering blood pressure

Answer 121:
A) Reducing proteinuria and slowing the progression of CKD

Explanation 121:
In CKD patients, ACE inhibitors primarily reduce proteinuria and slow the progression of CKD.

Question 122:
A 70-year-old patient with a history of heart failure is admitted with acute decompensated heart failure. On auscultation, the AG-ACNP hears crackles at the lung bases. What does this finding suggest?
A) Pleural effusion
B) Pneumonia

C) Pulmonary edema
D) Pneumothorax

Answer 122:
C) Pulmonary edema

Explanation 122:
Crackles at the lung bases on auscultation are indicative of pulmonary edema, a common finding in acute decompensated heart failure.

Question 123:
A geriatric patient with a history of falls is at risk for which common musculoskeletal injury?
A) Achilles tendon rupture
B) Rotator cuff tear
C) Vertebral compression fracture
D) Meniscal tear

Answer 123:
C) Vertebral compression fracture

Explanation 123:
Elderly patients with a history of falls are at risk for vertebral compression fractures, which can lead to back pain and loss of height.

Question 124:
A 72-year-old patient is admitted with acute shortness of breath and chest pain. On physical examination, a friction rub is heard during auscultation. What condition should the AG-ACNP suspect?
A) Myocardial infarction
B) Pneumothorax
C) Pericarditis
D) Pleurisy

Answer 124:
C) Pericarditis

Explanation 124:

The presence of a friction rub on auscultation is indicative of pericarditis, an inflammation of the pericardium that can cause chest pain and shortness of breath.

Question 125:
A geriatric patient with heart failure is prescribed a beta-blocker. What is the primary goal of beta-blocker therapy in the management of heart failure?
A) Reducing preload
B) Enhancing myocardial contractility
C) Blocking the effects of catecholamines
D) Dilating blood vessels

Answer 125:
C) Blocking the effects of catecholamines

Explanation 125:
The primary goal of beta-blocker therapy in the management of heart failure is to block the effects of catecholamines, reducing the workload of the heart.

Question 126:
A 74-year-old patient with a history of hypertension presents with acute-onset confusion, visual disturbances, and severe headache. On physical examination, blood pressure is significantly elevated. What is the most likely diagnosis?
A) Migraine with aura
B) Acute glaucoma
C) Hypertensive encephalopathy
D) Transient ischemic attack (TIA)

Answer 126:
C) Hypertensive encephalopathy

Explanation 126:
The combination of acute-onset confusion, visual disturbances, severe headache, and significantly elevated blood pressure is suggestive of hypertensive encephalopathy, a severe complication of hypertension.

Question 127:
A geriatric patient with a history of chronic kidney disease (CKD) is prescribed an angiotensin receptor blocker (ARB). What is the primary mechanism of action of ARBs in CKD patients?
A) Increasing serum creatinine levels
B) Enhancing renal sodium reabsorption
C) Dilating afferent arterioles
D) Reducing proteinuria and slowing the progression of CKD

Answer 127:
D) Reducing proteinuria and slowing the progression of CKD

Explanation 127:
In CKD patients, the primary mechanism of action of ARBs is to reduce proteinuria and slow the progression of CKD.

Question 128:
A geriatric patient with heart failure is prescribed an aldosterone antagonist. What is the primary mechanism of action of aldosterone antagonists in the management of heart failure?
A) Reducing preload
B) Enhancing myocardial contractility
C) Inhibiting the release of aldosterone
D) Increasing afterload

Answer 128:
C) Inhibiting the release of aldosterone

Explanation 128:
The primary mechanism of action of aldosterone antagonists in the management of heart failure is to inhibit the release of aldosterone, reducing sodium and water retention.

Question 129:
A geriatric patient with a history of falls is at risk for which common musculoskeletal injury?
A) Achilles tendon rupture
B) Rotator cuff tear
C) Vertebral compression fracture
D) Meniscal tear

Answer 129:
C) Vertebral compression fracture

Explanation 129:
Elderly patients with a history of falls are at risk for vertebral compression fractures, which can lead to back pain and loss of height.

Question 130:
A 74-year-old patient with a history of hypertension presents with sudden-onset chest pain, diaphoresis, and shortness of breath. On electrocardiogram (ECG), there are no ST-segment changes. What is the most likely diagnosis?
A) Non-ST-segment elevation myocardial infarction (NSTEMI)
B) Unstable angina
C) STEMI (ST-segment elevation myocardial infarction)
D) Stable angina

Answer 130:
B) Unstable angina

Explanation 130:
The absence of ST-segment changes on ECG in a patient with sudden-onset chest pain, diaphoresis, and shortness of breath is indicative of unstable angina.

Question 131:
A 68-year-old patient with a history of hypertension and diabetes presents with complaints of frequent urination, excessive thirst, and unexplained weight loss. What condition should the AG-ACNP suspect in this patient?
A) Hypertensive emergency
B) Diabetic ketoacidosis (DKA)
C) Hyperosmolar hyperglycemic state (HHS)
D) Hypoglycemia

Answer 131:
B) Diabetic ketoacidosis (DKA)

Explanation 131:

The patient's symptoms of frequent urination, excessive thirst, and unexplained weight loss are indicative of diabetic ketoacidosis (DKA), a serious complication of diabetes.

Question 132:

A geriatric patient with a history of chronic kidney disease (CKD) is prescribed an angiotensin-converting enzyme (ACE) inhibitor. What is the primary mechanism of action of ACE inhibitors in CKD patients?
A) Reducing proteinuria and slowing the progression of CKD
B) Enhancing renal sodium reabsorption
C) Dilating afferent arterioles
D) Lowering blood pressure

Answer 132:
A) Reducing proteinuria and slowing the progression of CKD

Explanation 132:
In CKD patients, ACE inhibitors primarily reduce proteinuria and slow the progression of CKD.

Question 133:

A 70-year-old patient with a history of heart failure is admitted with acute decompensated heart failure. On auscultation, the AG-ACNP hears crackles at the lung bases. What does this finding suggest?
A) Pleural effusion
B) Pneumonia
C) Pulmonary edema
D) Pneumothorax

Answer 133:
C) Pulmonary edema

Explanation 133:
Crackles at the lung bases on auscultation are indicative of pulmonary edema, a common finding in acute decompensated heart failure.

Question 134:
A geriatric patient with a history of falls is at risk for which common musculoskeletal injury?
A) Achilles tendon rupture
B) Rotator cuff tear
C) Vertebral compression fracture
D) Meniscal tear

Answer 134:
C) Vertebral compression fracture

Explanation 134:
Elderly patients with a history of falls are at risk for vertebral compression fractures, which can lead to back pain and loss of height.

Question 135:
A 72-year-old patient is admitted with acute shortness of breath and chest pain. On physical examination, a friction rub is heard during auscultation. What condition should the AG-ACNP suspect?
A) Myocardial infarction
B) Pneumothorax
C) Pericarditis
D) Pleurisy

Answer 135:
C) Pericarditis

Explanation 135:
The presence of a friction rub on auscultation is indicative of pericarditis, an inflammation of the pericardium that can cause chest pain and shortness of breath.

Question 136:
A geriatric patient with heart failure is prescribed a beta-blocker. What is the primary goal of beta-blocker therapy in the management of heart failure?
A) Reducing preload
B) Enhancing myocardial contractility
C) Blocking the effects of catecholamines
D) Dilating blood vessels

Answer 136:
C) Blocking the effects of catecholamines

Explanation 136:
The primary goal of beta-blocker therapy in the management of heart failure is to block the effects of catecholamines, reducing the workload of the heart.

Question 137:
A 74-year-old patient with a history of hypertension presents with sudden-onset chest pain, diaphoresis, and shortness of breath. On electrocardiogram (ECG), there are no ST-segment changes. What is the most likely diagnosis?
A) Migraine with aura
B) Acute glaucoma
C) Hypertensive encephalopathy
D) Transient ischemic attack (TIA)

Answer 137:
C) Hypertensive encephalopathy

Explanation 137:
The combination of acute-onset chest pain, diaphoresis, and shortness of breath, along with no ST-segment changes on ECG, is suggestive of hypertensive encephalopathy, a severe complication of hypertension.

Question 138:
A geriatric patient with a history of chronic kidney disease (CKD) is prescribed an angiotensin receptor blocker (ARB). What is the primary mechanism of action of ARBs in CKD patients?
A) Increasing serum creatinine levels
B) Enhancing renal sodium reabsorption
C) Dilating afferent arterioles
D) Reducing proteinuria and slowing the progression of CKD

Answer 138:
D) Reducing proteinuria and slowing the progression of CKD

Explanation 138:
In CKD patients, the primary mechanism of action of ARBs is to reduce proteinuria and slow the progression of CKD.

Question 139:
A geriatric patient with heart failure is prescribed an aldosterone antagonist. What is the primary mechanism of action of aldosterone antagonists in the management of heart failure?
A) Reducing preload
B) Enhancing myocardial contractility
C) Inhibiting the release of aldosterone
D) Increasing afterload

Answer 139:
C) Inhibiting the release of aldosterone

Explanation 139:
The primary mechanism of action of aldosterone antagonists in the management of heart failure is to inhibit the release of aldosterone, reducing sodium and water retention.

Question 140:
A geriatric patient with a history of falls is at risk for which common musculoskeletal injury?
A) Achilles tendon rupture
B) Rotator cuff tear
C) Vertebral compression fracture
D) Meniscal tear

Answer 140:
C) Vertebral compression fracture

Explanation 140:
Elderly patients with a history of falls are at risk for vertebral compression fractures, which can lead to back pain and loss of height.

Question 141:
A 74-year-old patient with a history of hypertension presents with sudden-onset chest pain, diaphoresis, and shortness of breath. On electrocardiogram (ECG), there are no ST-segment changes. What is the most likely diagnosis?
A) Non-ST-segment elevation myocardial infarction (NSTEMI)
B) Unstable angina
C) STEMI (ST-segment elevation myocardial infarction)
D) Stable angina

Answer 141:
B) Unstable angina

Explanation 141:
The absence of ST-segment changes on ECG in a patient with sudden-onset chest pain, diaphoresis, and shortness of breath is indicative of unstable angina.

Question 142:
A geriatric patient with a history of diabetes presents with symptoms of tingling and burning in the lower extremities. What complication of diabetes should the AG-ACNP suspect in this patient?
A) Diabetic retinopathy
B) Diabetic nephropathy
C) Diabetic neuropathy
D) Diabetic ketoacidosis

Answer 142:
C) Diabetic neuropathy

Explanation 142:
The symptoms of tingling and burning in the lower extremities are indicative of diabetic neuropathy, a common neurological complication of diabetes.

Question 143:
A 72-year-old patient is admitted with acute shortness of breath and chest pain. On physical examination, a friction rub is heard during auscultation. What condition should the AG-ACNP suspect?
A) Myocardial infarction
B) Pneumothorax
C) Pericarditis
D) Pleurisy

Answer 143:
C) Pericarditis

Explanation 143:
The presence of a friction rub on auscultation is indicative of pericarditis, an inflammation of the pericardium that can cause chest pain and shortness of breath.

Question 144:
A geriatric patient with heart failure is prescribed a beta-blocker. What is the primary goal of beta-blocker therapy in the management of heart failure?
A) Reducing preload
B) Enhancing myocardial contractility
C) Blocking the effects of catecholamines
D) Dilating blood vessels

Answer 144:
C) Blocking the effects of catecholamines

Explanation 144:
The primary goal of beta-blocker therapy in the management of heart failure is to block the effects of catecholamines, reducing the workload of the heart.

Question 145:
A 74-year-old patient with a history of hypertension presents with sudden-onset chest pain, diaphoresis, and shortness of breath. On electrocardiogram (ECG), there are no ST-segment changes. What is the most likely diagnosis?
A) Migraine with aura
B) Acute glaucoma
C) Hypertensive encephalopathy

D) Transient ischemic attack (TIA)

Answer 145:
C) Hypertensive encephalopathy

Explanation 145:
The combination of sudden-onset chest pain, diaphoresis, and no ST-segment changes on ECG is suggestive of hypertensive encephalopathy, a severe complication of hypertension.

Question 146:
A geriatric patient with a history of chronic kidney disease (CKD) is prescribed an angiotensin receptor blocker (ARB). What is the primary mechanism of action of ARBs in CKD patients?
A) Increasing serum creatinine levels
B) Enhancing renal sodium reabsorption
C) Dilating afferent arterioles
D) Reducing proteinuria and slowing the progression of CKD

Answer 146:
D) Reducing proteinuria and slowing the progression of CKD

Explanation 146:
In CKD patients, the primary mechanism of action of ARBs is to reduce proteinuria and slow the progression of CKD.

Question 147:
A geriatric patient with heart failure is prescribed an aldosterone antagonist. What is the primary mechanism of action of aldosterone antagonists in the management of heart failure?
A) Reducing preload
B) Enhancing myocardial contractility
C) Inhibiting the release of aldosterone
D) Increasing afterload

Answer 147:
C) Inhibiting the release of aldosterone

Explanation 147:

The primary mechanism of action of aldosterone antagonists in the management of heart failure is to inhibit the release of aldosterone, reducing sodium and water retention.

Question 148:
A geriatric patient with a history of falls is at risk for which common musculoskeletal injury?
A) Achilles tendon rupture
B) Rotator cuff tear
C) Vertebral compression fracture
D) Meniscal tear

Answer 148:
C) Vertebral compression fracture

Explanation 148:
Elderly patients with a history of falls are at risk for vertebral compression fractures, which can lead to back pain and loss of height.

Question 149:
A 74-year-old patient with a history of hypertension presents with sudden-onset chest pain, diaphoresis, and shortness of breath. On electrocardiogram (ECG), there are no ST-segment changes. What is the most likely diagnosis?
A) Non-ST-segment elevation myocardial infarction (NSTEMI)
B) Unstable angina
C) STEMI (ST-segment elevation myocardial infarction)
D) Stable angina

Answer 149:
B) Unstable angina

Explanation 149:
The absence of ST-segment changes on ECG in a patient with sudden-onset chest pain, diaphoresis, and shortness of breath is indicative of unstable angina.

Question 150:
A 68-year-old patient with a history of hypertension and diabetes presents with complaints of frequent urination, excessive thirst, and unexplained weight loss. What condition should the AG-ACNP suspect in this patient?
A) Hypertensive emergency
B) Diabetic ketoacidosis (DKA)
C) Hyperosmolar hyperglycemic state (HHS)
D) Hypoglycemia

Answer 150:
B) Diabetic ketoacidosis (DKA)

Explanation 150:
The patient's symptoms of frequent urination, excessive thirst, and unexplained weight loss are indicative of diabetic ketoacidosis (DKA), a serious complication of diabetes.

Question 151:
A geriatric patient with a history of chronic kidney disease (CKD) is prescribed an angiotensin-converting enzyme (ACE) inhibitor. What is the primary mechanism of action of ACE inhibitors in CKD patients?
A) Reducing proteinuria and slowing the progression of CKD
B) Enhancing renal sodium reabsorption
C) Dilating afferent arterioles
D) Lowering blood pressure

Answer 151:
A) Reducing proteinuria and slowing the progression of CKD

Explanation 151:
In CKD patients, ACE inhibitors primarily reduce proteinuria and slow the progression of CKD.

Question 152:
A 70-year-old patient with a history of heart failure is admitted with acute decompensated heart failure. On auscultation, the AG-ACNP hears crackles at the lung bases. What does this finding suggest?
A) Pleural effusion
B) Pneumonia
C) Pulmonary edema

D) Pneumothorax

Answer 152:
C) Pulmonary edema

Explanation 152:
Crackles at the lung bases on auscultation are indicative of pulmonary edema, a common finding in acute decompensated heart failure.

Question 153:
A geriatric patient with a history of falls is at risk for which common musculoskeletal injury?
A) Achilles tendon rupture
B) Rotator cuff tear
C) Vertebral compression fracture
D) Meniscal tear

Answer 153:
C) Vertebral compression fracture

Explanation 153:
Elderly patients with a history of falls are at risk for vertebral compression fractures, which can lead to back pain and loss of height.

Question 154:
A 72-year-old patient is admitted with acute shortness of breath and chest pain. On physical examination, a friction rub is heard during auscultation. What condition should the AG-ACNP suspect?
A) Myocardial infarction
B) Pneumothorax
C) Pericarditis
D) Pleurisy

Answer 154:
C) Pericarditis

Explanation 154:
The presence of a friction rub on auscultation is indicative of pericarditis, an inflammation of the pericardium that can cause chest pain and shortness of breath.

Question 155:
A geriatric patient with heart failure is prescribed a beta-blocker. What is the primary goal of beta-blocker therapy in the management of heart failure?
A) Reducing preload
B) Enhancing myocardial contractility
C) Blocking the effects of catecholamines
D) Dilating blood vessels

Answer 155:
C) Blocking the effects of catecholamines

Explanation 155:
The primary goal of beta-blocker therapy in the management of heart failure is to block the effects of catecholamines, reducing the workload of the heart.

Question 156:
A 74-year-old patient with a history of hypertension presents with sudden-onset chest pain, diaphoresis, and shortness of breath. On electrocardiogram (ECG), there are no ST-segment changes. What is the most likely diagnosis?
A) Migraine with aura
B) Acute glaucoma
C) Hypertensive encephalopathy
D) Transient ischemic attack (TIA)

Answer 156:
C) Hypertensive encephalopathy

Explanation 156:
The combination of sudden-onset chest pain, diaphoresis, and no ST-segment changes on ECG is suggestive of hypertensive encephalopathy, a severe complication of hypertension.

Question 157:
A geriatric patient with a history of chronic kidney disease (CKD) is prescribed an angiotensin receptor blocker (ARB). What is the primary mechanism of action of ARBs in CKD patients?
A) Increasing serum creatinine levels
B) Enhancing renal sodium reabsorption

C) Dilating afferent arterioles
D) Reducing proteinuria and slowing the progression of CKD

Answer 157:
D) Reducing proteinuria and slowing the progression of CKD

Explanation 157:
In CKD patients, the primary mechanism of action of ARBs is to reduce proteinuria and slow the progression of CKD.

Question 158:
A geriatric patient with heart failure is prescribed an aldosterone antagonist. What is the primary mechanism of action of aldosterone antagonists in the management of heart failure?
A) Reducing preload
B) Enhancing myocardial contractility
C) Inhibiting the release of aldosterone
D) Increasing afterload

Answer 158:
C) Inhibiting the release of aldosterone

Explanation 158:
The primary mechanism of action of aldosterone antagonists in the management of heart failure is to inhibit the release of aldosterone, reducing sodium and water retention.

Question 159:
A geriatric patient with a history of falls is at risk for which common musculoskeletal injury?
A) Achilles tendon rupture
B) Rotator cuff tear
C) Vertebral compression fracture
D) Meniscal tear

Answer 159:
C) Vertebral compression fracture

Explanation 159:

Elderly patients with a history of falls are at risk for vertebral compression fractures, which can lead to back pain and loss of height.

Question 160:

A 74-year-old patient with a history of hypertension presents with sudden-onset chest pain, diaphoresis, and shortness of breath. On electrocardiogram (ECG), there are no ST-segment changes. What is the most likely diagnosis?
A) Non-ST-segment elevation myocardial infarction (NSTEMI)
B) Unstable angina
C) STEMI (ST-segment elevation myocardial infarction)
D) Stable angina

Answer 160:
B) Unstable angina

Explanation 160:
The absence of ST-segment changes on ECG in a patient with sudden-onset chest pain, diaphoresis, and shortness of breath is indicative of unstable angina.

Question 161:

A geriatric patient with a history of diabetes presents with symptoms of tingling and burning in the lower extremities. What complication of diabetes should the AG-ACNP suspect in this patient?
A) Diabetic retinopathy
B) Diabetic nephropathy
C) Diabetic neuropathy
D) Diabetic ketoacidosis

Answer 161:
C) Diabetic neuropathy

Explanation 161:
The symptoms of tingling and burning in the lower extremities are indicative of diabetic neuropathy, a common neurological complication of diabetes.

Question 162:
A 72-year-old patient is admitted with acute shortness of breath and chest pain. On physical examination, a friction rub is heard during auscultation. What condition should the AG-ACNP suspect?
A) Myocardial infarction
B) Pneumothorax
C) Pericarditis
D) Pleurisy

Answer 162:
C) Pericarditis

Explanation 162:
The presence of a friction rub on auscultation is indicative of pericarditis, an inflammation of the pericardium that can cause chest pain and shortness of breath.

Question 163:
A geriatric patient with heart failure is prescribed a beta-blocker. What is the primary goal of beta-blocker therapy in the management of heart failure?
A) Reducing preload
B) Enhancing myocardial contractility
C) Blocking the effects of catecholamines
D) Dilating blood vessels

Answer 163:
C) Blocking the effects of catecholamines

Explanation 163:
The primary goal of beta-blocker therapy in the management of heart failure is to block the effects of catecholamines, reducing the workload of the heart.

Question 164:
A 74-year-old patient with a history of hypertension presents with sudden-onset chest pain, diaphoresis, and shortness of breath. On electrocardiogram (ECG), there are no ST-segment changes. What is the most likely diagnosis?
A) Migraine with aura
B) Acute glaucoma
C) Hypertensive encephalopathy

D) Transient ischemic attack (TIA)

Answer 164:
C) Hypertensive encephalopathy

Explanation 164:
The combination of sudden-onset chest pain, diaphoresis, and no ST-segment changes on ECG is suggestive of hypertensive encephalopathy, a severe complication of hypertension.

Question 165:
A geriatric patient with a history of chronic kidney disease (CKD) is prescribed an angiotensin receptor blocker (ARB). What is the primary mechanism of action of ARBs in CKD patients?
A) Increasing serum creatinine levels
B) Enhancing renal sodium reabsorption
C) Dilating afferent arterioles
D) Reducing proteinuria and slowing the progression of CKD

Answer 165:
D) Reducing proteinuria and slowing the progression of CKD

Explanation 165:
In CKD patients, the primary mechanism of action of ARBs is to reduce proteinuria and slow the progression of CKD.

Question 166:
A geriatric patient with heart failure is prescribed an aldosterone antagonist. What is the primary mechanism of action of aldosterone antagonists in the management of heart failure?
A) Reducing preload
B) Enhancing myocardial contractility
C) Inhibiting the release of aldosterone
D) Increasing afterload

Answer 166:
C) Inhibiting the release of aldosterone

Explanation 166:

The primary mechanism of action of aldosterone antagonists in the management of heart failure is to inhibit the release of aldosterone, reducing sodium and water retention.

Question 167:
A geriatric patient with a history of falls is at risk for which common musculoskeletal injury?
A) Achilles tendon rupture
B) Rotator cuff tear
C) Vertebral compression fracture
D) Meniscal tear

Answer 167:
C) Vertebral compression fracture

Explanation 167:
Elderly patients with a history of falls are at risk for vertebral compression fractures, which can lead to back pain and loss of height.

Question 168:
A 74-year-old patient with a history of hypertension presents with sudden-onset chest pain, diaphoresis, and shortness of breath. On electrocardiogram (ECG), there are no ST-segment changes. What is the most likely diagnosis?
A) Non-ST-segment elevation myocardial infarction (NSTEMI)
B) Unstable angina
C) STEMI (ST-segment elevation myocardial infarction)
D) Stable angina

Answer 168:
B) Unstable angina

Explanation 168:
The absence of ST-segment changes on ECG in a patient with sudden-onset chest pain, diaphoresis, and shortness of breath is indicative of unstable angina.

Question 169:
A geriatric patient with a history of diabetes presents with symptoms of tingling and burning in the lower extremities. What complication of diabetes should the AG-ACNP suspect in this patient?
A) Diabetic retinopathy
B) Diabetic nephropathy
C) Diabetic neuropathy
D) Diabetic ketoacidosis

Answer 169:
C) Diabetic neuropathy

Explanation 169:
The symptoms of tingling and burning in the lower extremities are indicative of diabetic neuropathy, a common neurological complication of diabetes.

Question 170:
A 72-year-old patient is admitted with acute shortness of breath and chest pain. On physical examination, a friction rub is heard during auscultation. What condition should the AG-ACNP suspect?
A) Myocardial infarction
B) Pneumothorax
C) Pericarditis
D) Pleurisy

Answer 170:
C) Pericarditis

Explanation 170:
The presence of a friction rub on auscultation is indicative of pericarditis, an inflammation of the pericardium that can cause chest pain and shortness of breath.

Question 171:
A geriatric patient with heart failure is prescribed a beta-blocker. What is the primary goal of beta-blocker therapy in the management of heart failure?
A) Reducing preload
B) Enhancing myocardial contractility
C) Blocking the effects of catecholamines
D) Dilating blood vessels

Answer 171:
C) Blocking the effects of catecholamines

Explanation 171:
The primary goal of beta-blocker therapy in the management of heart failure is to block the effects of catecholamines, reducing the workload of the heart.

Question 172:
A 74-year-old patient with a history of hypertension presents with sudden-onset chest pain, diaphoresis, and shortness of breath. On electrocardiogram (ECG), there are no ST-segment changes. What is the most likely diagnosis?
A) Migraine with aura
B) Acute glaucoma
C) Hypertensive encephalopathy
D) Transient ischemic attack (TIA)

Answer 172:
C) Hypertensive encephalopathy

Explanation 172:
The combination of sudden-onset chest pain, diaphoresis, and no ST-segment changes on ECG is suggestive of hypertensive encephalopathy, a severe complication of hypertension.

Question 173:
A geriatric patient with a history of chronic kidney disease (CKD) is prescribed an angiotensin receptor blocker (ARB). What is the primary mechanism of action of ARBs in CKD patients?
A) Increasing serum creatinine levels
B) Enhancing renal sodium reabsorption
C) Dilating afferent arterioles
D) Reducing proteinuria and slowing the progression of CKD

Answer 173:
D) Reducing proteinuria and slowing the progression of CKD

Explanation 173:

In CKD patients, the primary mechanism of action of ARBs is to reduce proteinuria and slow the progression of CKD.

Question 174:
A geriatric patient with heart failure is prescribed an aldosterone antagonist. What is the primary mechanism of action of aldosterone antagonists in the management of heart failure?
A) Reducing preload
B) Enhancing myocardial contractility
C) Inhibiting the release of aldosterone
D) Increasing afterload

Answer 174:
C) Inhibiting the release of aldosterone

Explanation 174:
The primary mechanism of action of aldosterone antagonists in the management of heart failure is to inhibit the release of aldosterone, reducing sodium and water retention.

Question 175:
A geriatric patient with a history of falls is at risk for which common musculoskeletal injury?
A) Achilles tendon rupture
B) Rotator cuff tear
C) Vertebral compression fracture
D) Meniscal tear

Answer 175:
C) Vertebral compression fracture

Explanation 175:
Elderly patients with a history of falls are at risk for vertebral compression fractures, which can lead to back pain and loss of height.

Question 176:
A 74-year-old patient with a history of hypertension presents with sudden-onset chest pain, diaphoresis, and shortness of breath. On electrocardiogram (ECG), there are no ST-segment changes. What is the most likely diagnosis?
A) Non-ST-segment elevation myocardial infarction (NSTEMI)
B) Unstable angina
C) STEMI (ST-segment elevation myocardial infarction)
D) Stable angina

Answer 176:
B) Unstable angina

Explanation 176:
The absence of ST-segment changes on ECG in a patient with sudden-onset chest pain, diaphoresis, and shortness of breath is indicative of unstable angina.

Question 177:
A geriatric patient with a history of diabetes presents with symptoms of tingling and burning in the lower extremities. What complication of diabetes should the AG-ACNP suspect in this patient?
A) Diabetic retinopathy
B) Diabetic nephropathy
C) Diabetic neuropathy
D) Diabetic ketoacidosis

Answer 177:
C) Diabetic neuropathy

Explanation 177:
The symptoms of tingling and burning in the lower extremities are indicative of diabetic neuropathy, a common neurological complication of diabetes.

uestion 178:

A 72-year-old patient is admitted with acute shortness of breath and chest pain. On physical examination, a friction rub is heard during auscultation. What condition should the AG-ACNP suspect?

A) Myocardial infarction

B) Pneumothorax

C) Pericarditis

D) Pleurisy

Answer 178:

C) Pericarditis

Explanation 178:

The presence of a friction rub on auscultation is indicative of pericarditis, an inflammation of the pericardium that can cause chest pain and shortness of breath.

Question 179:

A geriatric patient with heart failure is prescribed a beta-blocker. What is the primary goal of beta-blocker therapy in the management of heart failure?

A) Reducing preload

B) Enhancing myocardial contractility

C) Blocking the effects of catecholamines

D) Dilating blood vessels

Answer 179:

C) Blocking the effects of catecholamines

Explanation 179:

The primary goal of beta-blocker therapy in the management of heart failure is to block the effects of catecholamines, reducing the workload of the heart.

Question 180:

A 74-year-old patient with a history of hypertension presents with sudden-onset chest pain, diaphoresis, and shortness of breath. On electrocardiogram (ECG), there are no ST-segment changes. What is the most likely diagnosis?

A) Migraine with aura
B) Acute glaucoma
C) Hypertensive encephalopathy
D) Transient ischemic attack (TIA)

Answer 180:
C) Hypertensive encephalopathy

Explanation 180:
The combination of sudden-onset chest pain, diaphoresis, and no ST-segment changes on ECG is suggestive of hypertensive encephalopathy, a severe complication of hypertension.